THE WAY OF FIVE

The Body in Balance

David Schultz, M.D.

outskirts press
DENVER, COLORADO

The opinions expressed in this manuscript are solely the opinions of the author and do not represent the opinions or thoughts of the publisher. The author has represented and warranted full ownership and/or legal right to publish all the materials in this book.

The Way of Five
The Body in Balance
All Rights Reserved.
Copyright © 2015 David Schultz, M.D.
v3.0

Cover Photo © 2015 thinkstockphotos.com. Interior Illustrations by Laura Barnhardt Corle.
All rights reserved - used with permission.

This book may not be reproduced, transmitted, or stored in whole or in part by any means, including graphic, electronic, or mechanical without the express written consent of the publisher except in the case of brief quotations embodied in critical articles and reviews.

Outskirts Press, Inc.
http://www.outskirtspress.com

ISBN: 978-1-4787-2714-9

Outskirts Press and the "OP" logo are trademarks belonging to Outskirts Press, Inc.

PRINTED IN THE UNITED STATES OF AMERICA

1
Patterns

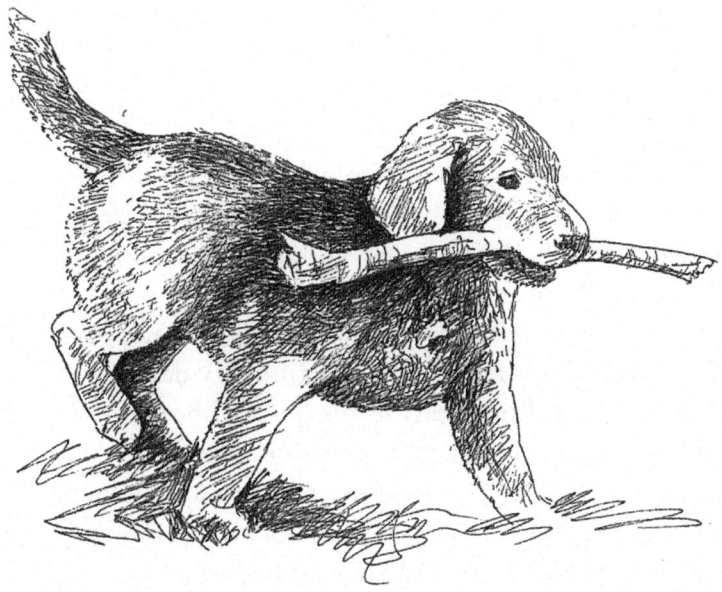

My Grandfather leaned against his workbench and brushed aside some wood shavings. Pouring coffee from a battered thermos, he started his " nutrition" speech.

"You are what you eat," he said as he put the thermos bottle back in its spot.

I didn't really want to hear that speech so I picked up a complex pattern off the workbench and started to fidget with it. I started running my fingers over the filleted groove between two larger sections.

"I feel great every day," he said.

"No aches or pains, no arthritis in my fingers."

He held up his eighty-year-old fingers for inspection. They certainly were straight and strong, although the skin was starting to get a bit thin.

"I sleep good, I eat good, my bowels move every day. Nobody has it any better than me…" My grandfather always was grateful for the little blessings of life.

I took the wooden sculpture and started to lightly toss it up and down. I knew that this would abbreviate his "health talk."

He looked at me.

"I just spent forty hours on that."

I knew that he had…impossibilities of wooden curves glistening with a quaint shellac peculiar to the pattern maker's trade.

"You can't expect a body to run on just cigarettes and coffee for breakfast."

I agreed and mentally started to tick off the ingredients of his daily breakfast for the past thirty years-- a bowl of raisin bran or shredded wheat, topped with bananas and about three tablespoons of wheat germ sprinkled on top with milk.

"I don't mean to tell you what to do, David, but a person could do a lot worse than to eat a little wheat germ every day."

We look forward five years to his hospital bed, where he recuperated a few hours after a cataract operation. He had an internist check him over while there as his blood pressure was a bit high.

"He gave me a prescription for high blood pressure pills and wants to see me in his office in two weeks," he said.

I knew at the age of eighty-five he wasn't about to start taking pills of any kind as it was an article of faith in our house that he hadn't done so for fifty years.

Grampa chuckled, "I suppose he thinks he'll have a new customer."

At the age of one hundred, my grandfather had a stroke. He said, "When the time comes, don't prolong it! One hundred years old is old enough!"

His legs had given out. His mind was perfect. He demanded cold orange juice and potato chips, no thickener. He choked two weeks later, eating what he wanted, and he died.

Twenty years later, I know now that much of my clinical diagnostic inquiry day to day, starts with *his* review of the body's functions:

sleeping, walking, eliminating, eating. It's pretty simple really. All the systems should work pretty well and one should feel well every day.

The Five Questions I ask my patients are these --

Do you sleep well each night and feel refreshed in the morning?

Do you eat well and enjoy your meals? Is your weight stable?

Do you move your bowels easily every day?

Can you walk a mile? Can you get all your work done?

Are you cheerful and productive every day?

These questions are five **gateways** for further inquiry. A negative response to any one of them may indicate significant or even serious disease. Just as a wooden pattern must conform to its designer's specification, the functions of the body should come up to specs as well.

Now, in 2015, our culture, and the health of the nation has degenerated significantly since the first edition of this book. Autoimmune diseases such as rheumatoid arthritis and lupus are rising. Autism is skyrocketing. Cancer has overtaken heart disease as the number one killer in the elderly. The importance of good food, clean water and exercise is more important than ever to fight the chemical pollutants, job and social stresses, and electromagnetic waves that are filling our world.

Ask yourself THE FIVE QUESTIONS, see what the answers are...

2
Sleeping...

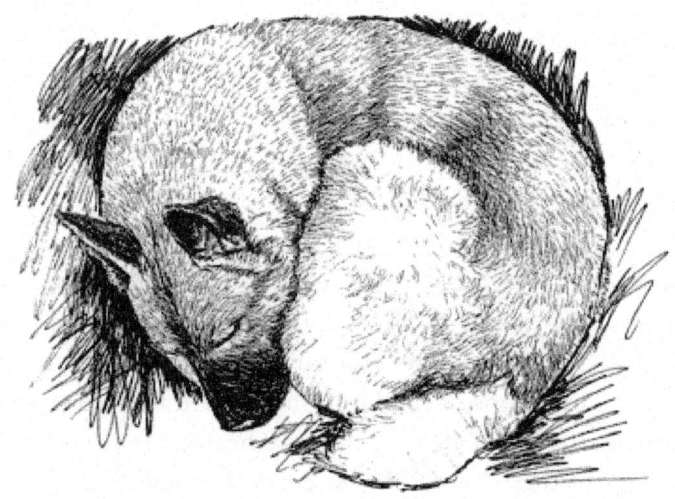

Do You Sleep Well Each Night And Feel Refreshed In The Morning?

Even last night and two nights more I lay,
I couldn't win thee, Sleep! By any stealth
So do not let me wear tonight away

Without Thee, what is all the morning's wealth
Come, Blessed barrier between day and day

SLEEPING...

Dear Mother of freshest thoughts and joyous health!
William Wordsworth from "To Sleep"

I'm sure these words written two hundred years ago are just as true today. Sleep is the one third of life which prepares us for the rest. Little productive thought or work is accomplished without proper sleep.

I remember vividly my residency days, working all day, being sleep-deprived all night, and trying to do responsible work the next day. It was a pretty tough balancing act I assure you. I recall falling asleep during surgery holding some dumb retractor...good thing my sub-conscious mind was clever enough to keep me from pitching forward into the patient's abdominal cavity and rupturing a bunch of organs. That never happened though; I was a good sleep walker -- or more correctly a good sleep stander.

Medical science is just now starting to inquire as to the nature of sleep problems, and also recognize their great importance.

Insomnia is a general term for when we don't sleep well. There are primary sleep disorders, types of insomnia, parasomnias, and other such things, intricate in nature, and poorly understood. Far more frequently, sleep is disturbed by a disease or disorder of another organ system, be it the heart, the lungs, the joints, or the urinary system.

Sleep apnea

Sleep apnea is one of the most under-diagnosed disorders in America today. Some studies suggest 7-8% of Caucasian seniors (over 65) and nearly twice that rate of African-Americans suffer from this problem. Some authors estimate that 90 percent of sleep apnea is not diagnosed!

Airway problems cause snoring and partial or almost complete obstruction of the airway when the sleep apnea sufferer lies down. The apnea part is when the person actually stops breathing. They usually start up again with a loud snort and often wake their bedmates or themselves. So often, I diagnose this disorder by the reports of spouses who lie awake at night alternately being rattled by the noisy snoring or wondering if the sufferer is going to take another breath.

This disorder leads to all kinds of health problems -- they include:
- chronic fatigue
- daytime drowsiness
- confusion and listlessness
- memory problems
- high blood pressure
- depression

All these serious maladies arise because the poor patient is chronically sleep deprived. The following case study illustrates the dramatic improvement possible following diagnosis and treatment.

M.D. was a sixty-year-old woman who suffered from extreme obesity, hypertension, and uncontrolled diabetes. At well over three hundred pounds, her diabetes was out of control, her feet hurt, her blood pressure was out of control, and she felt horrible. About two years ago, she underwent sleep study analysis which showed her to be suffering from severe sleep apnea. She stopped breathing for up to 45 seconds at a time and had dozens of apnea spells throughout thenight. She was fitted with a CPAP machine to provide continuous pressure in the back of her throat to keep the tissues from collapsing and blocking her airway. She announced that she felt immediately better with marked increase in energy and daytime alertness. I saw the patient two months later and she had lost twenty pounds without really trying. At the end of one year, she had lost nearly a hundred pounds, I was able to discontinue all of her blood pressure medicines and she was no longer diabetic! Interestingly, this patient never went on a diet, and never undertook any real exercise program. She was just awake much more and felt like doing more activity during the day!

Sleep apnea is a very sneaky disorder in that there is a point of no return.... where a person cannot overcome it by themselves. As they become more and more fatigued and experience more daytime sleepiness, their ability to exercise and lose weight declines. They gain more weight, and their necks become fatter with even less room for the airway. It is a true vicious cycle.

Sleep apnea causes marked daytime sleepiness and is a common cause of traffic accidents. European studies show that drowsiness causes up to 30% of accidents. Here in the U.S., the percentage of accidents due to sleepiness would be much less because we are so lax on drunk driving. It is still a huge problem!

Much of high blood pressure problems may be due to sleep apnea. Recent articles are suggesting a very strong association between the two disorders. Physicians need to start asking pointed questions regarding quality of sleep, daytime drowsiness, snoring habits and examining the palates and airways of patients with sleep apnea in mind.

Losing weight helps. However, it is so, so hard to do when one feels so tired, and lacks ambition to exercise. I usually recommend a CPAP (continuous positive airway pressure) machine while the patient loses weight and encourage them to view it as temporary. Once the patient loses weight and reduces his neck size, perhaps the machine can be retired again.

Palate remodeling surgery sometimes is recommended to enlarge the posterior pharynx. It usually does not help. I usually recommend a trial of CPAP first. Often the patient will say, "I feel great, I don't need any surgery" then the matter is finished. If the patient feels the hassle of using the machine is too burdensome, then they can go and have the re-shaping done.

Sleep apnea is not a rare disorder. Quite to the contrary! I have diagnosed literally hundreds of patients in the past ten years who were suffering and now have much more energy!

New research suggests that sleep apnea will change the biochemistry of the patient, in that inflammatory chemicals are increased. This may help explain why coronary disease is increased in the sleep apnea sufferer.

GERD - Gastroesophageal Reflux Disease

This disorder occurs when the valve at the top of the stomach doesn't stay shut tight enough, allowing food and stomach contents to come back up. This usually happens most severely at night when the patient is lying down and trying to sleep. The sleep of the GERD sufferer is interrupted by heartburn rising into the chest. Occasionally the stomach acid will go all the way up to the larynx and cause an unpleasant fit of choking after inhaling some stomach juice (!)

Sometime the patient is not aware of the refluxing at all. This can be an aggravating factor in asthma and chronic hoarseness. Often the vocal cords will be red from the acid coming backwards.

This disorder is strongly associated with obesity. The corpulent abdomen rests on the anatomical stomach and distorts the architecture of the valve at the top. Nonetheless, many non-obese patients suffer from this as well.... and even some very lean ones.

Doctors and patients need to be aware that some medicines aggravate this problem by relaxing the valve at the top of the stomach. Most notorious are the blood pressure medicines, the calcium channel blockers (Cardizem, Adalat, Procardia, Tizac, and all their generic equivalents).

Antidepressants that have anticholinergic side effects (Elavil, Desyrl, Imipramine), and bladder drugs (Ditropan) aggravate GERD and should be used with caution. Paradoxically, sleep aids in the Valium (benzodiazepines) family can do this also; working against the purpose it was prescribed.

Many simple things can be done to alleviate the nocturnal symptoms of GERD.

Eating small meals -not distending the stomach, particularly before retiring will help most every GERD sufferer.

Losing weight - There is very strong correlation between obesity and acid reflux. A fat abdomen pushes on the stomach and causes increased positive pressure to allow stomach contents to go backwards.

SLEEPING...

The snorting and struggling associated with sleep apnea (see previous section) can also create negative pressure in the chest and cause acid to flow backwards. Sometimes treating sleep apnea can vastly help GERD as well!

Elevate the bed by using blocks under the bed or, much better, use a bed wedge to raise the mattress. It works much better than simply piling up pillows and trying to stay on them. Simple antacids at bedtime - a tablespoon of Maalox at bedtime will work for many people. New proton pump inhibitors (PPIs) such as Prilosec, and Nexium work very well; however, it is better to address underlying causes than take pills for something correctable.

Unfortunately, acid reflux is not a benign disorder. After a time, changes at the esophageal-stomach junction can cause scarring (food sticking when you swallow?) and even cancer. These people will need to have the stomach and esophagus looked at directly and biopsied with a flexible scope.

Some people will require a potent drug like Prilosec or Prevacid for long term control, however these drugs too have their problems.

Urinary problems and sleep

Getting up from bed every couple of hours to urinate can be a problem for both men and women. Usually not serious, this can be a detriment to quality of life.

For the man

Men's problems center around the prostate gland, causing poor emptying of the bladder and chronic sensations of fullness. The prostate is a walnut-sized gland, which lies between the bladder and the penis. It acts as a junction where water, sugars, and volume are added to seminal fluid before exiting the urethra. Prostatic hypertrophy is one of the most common ailments, affecting almost every man over the age of sixty to a greater or lesser degree.

Every man over the age of forty should have a digital prostate exam yearly to check for prostate cancer. One of the great myths is that the new PSA blood test takes the place of the digital rectal exam to detect prostate cancer. It does not! About 85% of prostate cancers cause the body to create PSA, leaving a full 15% not covered at all. Not my kind of odds at all. As unpleasant as it is, the old fashioned "finger wave" is necessary to detect lumps in the prostate which could turn out to be cancer.

Benign Prostatic Hypertrophy or BPH is an extremely common disorder, in which a non-cancerous, but enlarged, prostate obstructs the urethra. The symptoms produced are -- poor stream, dribbling, sensations of chronic bladder fullness, and frequent urination. In severe cases, the flow is markedly impaired and the man may become prone to urinary infections.

Studies exist in the scientific literature, which, if one digs a little, suggest that diet can have an effect on the stimulation and growth of the prostate. Saxe et al. showed in a small study where men had undergone prostatectomy for prostate cancer that a low fat, plant based diet markedly slowed the rise in PSA levels over controls. Other studies show low fat diets with omega three oil supplementation have a significant effect on the aggressiveness of a prostate tumor upon resection.

There are drugs available which are fairly effective in reducing the size of the prostate, increasing flow and benefitting sleep. When these fail, there is always the TURP, or trans-urethral resection of the prostate, to surgically open a wider channel.

Women's problems

Women's urinary problems affecting sleep are usually a function of the health of the bladder -- its tone, its shape (fallen?) and the health of the sphincter muscle leading out of the bladder to keep the urine in place. Fallen bladder or bladder prolapse is an extremely common affliction in women who have had children.

This distorts the normal shape of the bladder, making the fallen or dependant section more cone-shaped and less round and capacious. This gives sensations of bladder fullness as the narrowed area becomes full with urine; one has to go to the bathroom before the whole bladder space can be utilized. The falling bladder can also put traction on the tissue next to the urethral sphincter decreasing its effectiveness in squeezing and holding the urine in place.

If the falling is not too severe, squeezing exercises (Kegel exercises) can increase the strength of the pelvic floor where the urethra passes through and helps with urinary incontinence. These are accomplished by trying to reproduce the feeling of squeezing off the urine (no hands, ladies!) This will strengthen the muscle of the pelvic floor giving important support to all the organs there, controlling urinary and fecal incontinence as well.

Interstitial cystitis

Interstitial cystitis is a mysterious disorder, which involves a chronic inflammation of the bladder wall. Most sufferers have been to numerous physicians and treated for many, many urinary infections before the true nature of the disorder becomes apparent. When the urine is examined microscopically, pus is seen but bacteria is not -- thus the patient has inflammation but not infection. The sum of this action is that the bladder wall is irritated and is prone to muscular spasms resulting in urgency to urinate and frequently painful intercourse (the posterior bladder and anterior vagina sharing a thin wall separating the two organs).

This disorder is so frustrating that it is frequently featured in women's magazines, usually with the title "The Disease Your Doctor Will Miss" or something equally dreadful. Indeed the average woman sees something like nineteen different doctors before diagnosis is made. But even then, they don't have it right...

I believe that interstitial cystitis is an inflammatory disorder with an allergic basis. There is much data to support this:

Allergic bladder symptoms have been reported in the literature for decades. Patients who suffer from interstitial cystitis also have more classic allergies such as pollinosis to ragweed and tree pollen. These patients also have an increased incidence of irritable bowel syndrome, suggesting food intolerances and allergies.

On electron microscopy, many of the mast cells located in the bladder wall are activated in interstitial cystitis sufferers. These are the same cells which cause problems in ragweed sufferers when their nose drips and itches. Urine samples from these patients likewise have shown to contain elevated levels of histamine metabolites which are released from the mast cell granules when stimulated.

What could be the likely triggers for this? The most likely culprits in this disorder are food fragments and attached antibodies (antigen-antibody complexes) which are filtered through the kidney and then lie in the bladder causing the reactions.

Sufferers from interstitial cystitis should have a trial of an elimination diet to see if there are ingested food fractions which are exciting an inflammatory response in the bladder wall. The best foods to eliminate at first are: cow's milk, wheat and flour products, corn products, egg, yeast and artificial sweeteners and colorings. If any of these are responsible, symptoms should resolve in about a week.

(See the Cave Man Diet in the "Moving" chapter.)

Diabetes and sleep

Frequent nighttime urination may be a sign of diabetes, and diabetes is an epidemic which is plaguing the nation right now! Anyone getting up from bed to urinate more than once a night should be checked for diabetes.

More completely covered in the section on moving and obesity, diabetes is one of the most pressing public health issues in America today.

Depression and sleep

Although covered more fully in the section on the mind, sleep disturbance is a cardinal symptom of depression. Most depressed people have sleep disturbance: either too much or too little or not at the right time.

The classic case is the person with early morning wakening (EMW)–the inability to stay asleep through the night. Typically, the depressed person falls asleep OK, then awakens early in the morning say 3:00 or 4:00 A.M. They have great difficulty in falling back to sleep. If they do, they typically feel bad in the AM when it's time to get up and get going.

Others have trouble falling asleep at bedtime. This is a common variant which affects as many as 20-30% of depressed persons. These people sometimes benefit more from sedating antidepressants given at bedtime to aid in the falling asleep process.

Some depressed people sleep too much instead of too little -- they experience hyper-somnolence. As a result of depression they are sleeping many hours a day yet have no energy.

So common is sleep disorder in depression that it always must be considered along with the other causes of disordered sleep.

Restless leg syndrome

Many people find it difficult to fall asleep when first supine because their legs hurt. Not always a pain exactly, the sensation is frequently a creeping sensation, a tingling, a burning and often just an urgency to wiggle the legs. Thus, sleep comes hard to the sufferer of this disorder.

The cause of restless leg syndrome is unknown, but there are some clues as we approach the subject obliquely. We know that the condition usually occurs in older adults, and rarely in children and adolescents. Pregnant women suffer from this disorder yet never had it before pregnancy and never have it after they deliver. Scientific papers involving pregnant women are intriguing and iron and/or folate deficiency are implicated as suspected culprits.

Treatments for restless leg syndrome are usually directed toward the nervous system though I strongly doubt that is where the basic problem lies. Valium and related drugs (Clonazapam) work very well in eliminating the problem, yet that causes problems of addiction, morning grogginess and is expensive. I doubt if these patients are suffering from a Clonazapam deficiency. The more recent trend is to use Parkinson's type drugs to stimulate the dopamine system in the brain.

The large numbers of people suffering from this disorder (15%

by some sources) would seem to go against a genetic hypothesis. Yet, many authors postulate a defect in dopamine metabolism. I would like to offer a toxic hypothesis in that perhaps the aging brains of restless legs symptom sufferers have received a common insult to some of the dopamine- containing areas resulting in the findings now in vogue. Thus, the brain findings are really the result of another insult rather than a first cause of the condition.

Restless leg syndrome is an extremely common cause of insomnia and its basic root cause is unknown. I feel it is worth using whatever treatment works in that the morbidity of the condition does cause significant problems in quality of life in terms of fatigue, depression, and poor cognitive performance during the waking hours.

Congestive heart failure

Sometimes heart failure can first be detected through sleep disturbance. This typically comes to light when the patient complains, "they can no longer lie flat in bed." Occasionally, they will awaken with a start when they have fallen off the pillows that they have piled up. This situation can arise more insidiously, perhaps with a viral infection of the heart. Usually this type of patient will complain of leg swelling during the daytime and decreased ability to walk briskly. But, just as often, they come to a doctor because they are not sleeping well.

Shift working bad for health

I know a lot of people who work on third shift (11:00 P.M. to 7:00 A.M. and its variants) and I try to encourage them to get off if possible. Many scientific studies show that trying to work at night and sleep during the day is bad for health.

Before I went to medical school, I worked eleven to seven in a carborundum factory. I went to bed at 8:00 A.M., slept for a few hours, would usually get up around 1:00 P.M. because I couldn't sleep very well, did a few chores, went to bed again at 7:00, tried to sleep a little more and then went in to work. I was chronically tired all the time. I hated it.

SLEEPING...

Many studies show that night workers suffer poorer health than day workers in all kinds of ways.

They are prone to more hypertension, more depression, more accidents and weaker immune systems leading to flu and colds. The circadian (from the Latin *circa* [around] and *dies* [day]) rhythms of the day and night are dictated by the cycles of the sunlight and darkness. Your body has circadian rhythms as well which are geared to the light and darkness surrounding you. I do have patients who have worked at night for years, and even decades, without apparent harm. Some people get used to it -

- I don't think I ever could.

Sleep disturbances are very real, very common, and very serious detriments to health. As I have shown, they often contribute to other serious problems such as hypertension, accidents, and depression in a chain reaction of events. If one does not feel well rested after sleeping, there is probably something significantly wrong. It is worth investigating.

3

Eating

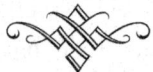

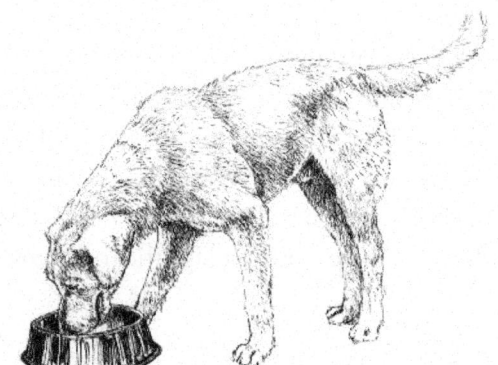

Do You Eat Your Meals With a Good Appetite? Is Your Weight Stable?

A sick dog won't eat.
-old saying

As I helped the old lady up onto the exam table, I glanced over to her chart and list of medications. I quickly counted nine different prescription drugs: medications for hypertension, arthritis, thyroid, Parkinson's disease, antidepressants and drugs for stomach acid reflux. I asked her,
"How is your appetite?"
"Too good!" she chuckled.

EATING

Even though this lady (at over eighty years of age) had many medical problems, I knew she was still generally "OK." Everything was more or less stable.

By that one positive reply I knew that her heart was probably good, she wasn't in kidney failure nor did she have cancer.

This is the briefest of all sections. A person whose appetite is poor is sick, and the list of maladies responsible is not too terribly long.

Bugs in your stomach - Helicobacter Pylori

In 1982 Australian researchers Barry Marshall and Robin Warren theorized that stomach ulcers were caused by bacterial infection, not from stress or coffee or other traditional culprits.[1] They chose the time-honored method of self-inoculation. They infected themselves with the suspected agent and Voila! - a nice stomach ulcer followed. The Helicobacter Pylori connection is another example of what one learned in medical school being wrong twenty years later.

The infection of helicobacter pylori (hereafter known as H, pylori) in the stomach causes a wide spectrum of discomfort[2]. From the large eroding ulcer, to excessive gas and belching, to vague burning sensations, the presence of this bug can cause them all. I have been impressed with the range of symptoms that can be banished with the appropriate course of antibiotics. Studies have shown that 90% of patients suffering from duodenal ulcers and 60% of gastric ulcers (in the stomach) are colonized with this bacterium.

Children are not immune from this disorder. A 1994 French study showed that a high percentage of children being evaluated for abdominal pain had this bacteria !

Abdominal pain in children is always a challenging diagnostic problem, so a simple screen for elevated antibodies against this bacteria or a breath test for their metabolites would seem a helpful step toward diagnosis.

---

1   Marshall B.J., Warren J.R., "Unidentified Curve Bacilli in the Stomach of Patients with Gastritis and Peptic Ulceration" Lancet 1984 Jun 16: (8390): 1311-5
2   Pakodi F, Et al, " Helicobacter Pylori One Bacterium and a broad spectrum of Human Disease ! An Overview " *J Physio Paris.*, 2000 Mar-Apr;94(2):139-52

Cycles of disease

I recently checked top medications prescribed for the year 2013 and right up there at number two was Nexium, a potent (and very expensive) acid blocker. This drug reduces the production of hydrochloric acid in the stomach for long periods of time. I frequently run across patients who have been on this drug for years and I have to ask myself, "What is it that makes these people's stomachs hurt for so long?" - Will they have to be on these drugs forever?"[3]

Here is one possible chain of events:

Bad habits (cigarettes and booze) lead to ... cell injury of the stomach lining ... to infection with H. pylori ... to increased susceptibility to acid injury ... to gastritis and ulcers.

Interestingly, people who take these acid (proton pump inhibitors) blockers rarely get off them. It is my experience that people who become infected with H. pylori once will get re-infected again. (Same family? Same bad habits? Same house? Same cat? Who knows?) I wonder if they feel that they can get away with more and not have their stomach hurt. So why would one not take them?

I can offer one simple theory -- If the stomach is injured, reducing the amount of acid there will certainly cause less burning sensation. But won't that allow the person to continue their bad habits until a cancer finally forms in the stomach or esophagus? I have to think that the continued need for acid blockers indicates a continued unhealthy process in the stomach, be it toxic exposure, allergic reactions, nicotine poisoning, H. pylori infection, or some other yet to be discovered imbalance that their doctor has yet to find.

One interesting side effect of these potent drugs is that surgery for stomach ulcers is a minuscule fraction of what it was thirty years ago. Many surgical interns go their whole training period without doing a stomach resection for peptic ulcers or a vagotomy. That part is good (I think).

---

[3] Hurenkamp GJ, et al. "Arrest of CHronic Acid Suppression Drug use After Successful Helicobacter pylori Eradication in Patient with Peptic ulcer Disease: A six Month Follow- up Study" *Alimen Pharmacol Ther*, 20001 Jul; 15(7) ;1047-54

Cancer, cancer, and more cancer

Cancers kill the appetite, sometimes in early stages. They release strange toxins with exotic names such as Cadaverin and Putrifactant. The nomenclature man knew what he was about.

The vast majority of my patients overeat, and when one presents with a dropping weight without reason, it is certainly cause for alarm. Gastrointestinal cancers seem to have a particular affinity for killing the appetite, particularly the desire for meats. Cancer of the colon occurs when the regulatory mechanism of the cells go haywire and start to replicate uncontrolled. With any luck, the cells will take on the form of an exophytic (out-growing) form, develop into an unstable, gangling mess and will bleed early on in the process. This will alert patient and physician to the problem and the cancer can be removed early and permanently. The less fortunate patient will develop an in-growing type of cancer that doesn't bleed into the stool. These are usually discovered much later and woe to the patient.

Cancers of the esophagus and stomach often present late with little disturbance of the eating process for some time. Epidemiological studies have shown that consumption of smoked meats, pickled stuff and the usual cigarettes and booze are strong carcinogens in this area. Cancer of the stomach used to be far more common, ostensibly due to a reduction of smoked, salted, and preserved meats in our American diet.

The rest of the cancers also affect the appetite but not so reliably as those of the stomach and bowel. Breast cancer, lung cancer, reproductive cancers and lymphatic cancers all cause anorexia, but so often, too late in the process to be any warning.

The NIH gets one right...cancer is environmental, (mostly)

About fifteen years ago, the National Institute of Health made a pronouncement- that 90% of cancers were due to what we ate, smoked, inhaled and drank. In other words, our exposure to our environment has a lot to do with whether we get cancer.

However, we have all seen families where cancer runs deep and long. Colon cancer and pancreatic cancer are two that seem to have definite family tendencies.

The most reasonable explanation to me is that many cancers result from a combination of genetic predisposition and environmental triggers.

All cancers involve defects in the genetic machinery of the cells controlling replication. Otherwise, those cells would behave themselves and not replicate madly into piled up gobs of murder. Patients may inherit a tendency toward cancer from their parents, then trigger the cells to grow wildly by further bungling up the DNA...by inhaling and ingesting bad stuff.

Members of families inherit more than just their genetic material. They share the same living spaces and exposure to asbestos and radon and other chemicals. They share the same dietary habits (or dietary bad habits!) and thus, expose themselves to many of the same toxins and problems.

It doesn't surprise me that colon cancer runs in families...most members learn to eat the same way for the first eighteen years of their lives, and if it is a chronically low fiber diet, the whole family is in store for bowel problems.

Cardiac cachexia

This is not an entry symptom like the rest but is included to demonstrate a point -- disease in one major organ system can cause severe disturbance in another. To be cachexic means to be skeletal, a condition of extreme wasting. When the heart is failing, it has little capacity to spare. Eating and digesting food requires blood flow to be shunted to the stomach for it to perform its churning and mixing functions. A person may experience abdominal discomfort after a meal when their degree of heart function is badly diminished and there is no blood supply to spare.

Severely decreased lung function can cause a similar syndrome when the work of breathing becomes so severe it interferes with eating. Patients with emphysema in its end stages are typically very thin, finding it hard to chew and swallow when they are working so hard.

EATING

Anorexia and nausea and acute disease

Sir Zachary Cope in his classic book <u>The Early Diagnosis of the Acute Abdomen</u> said regarding acute appendicitis - "If the patient is hungry you'd best think of another diagnosis!" The appetite being a very sensitive indicator of disease, or distress of the alimentary tract, from top to bottom.

This one phrase or aphorism has helped me repeatedly through the past twenty years, even though it was written in 1922. I will relate the following interesting case...

B.R. was a 19-year-old boy who came to the office one afternoon with a belly ache. His distress had started the day before with vague feelings of nausea and unease. He developed pain centered around his belly button during the night, and by the time I saw him, it had shifted to the right lower quadrant. I called a surgeon and had the boy go over to his office for further examination. Five hours later, after my office had closed, I called the hospital to see how the lad was doing. I found out that he was in radiology getting a CAT scan of the abdomen. The boy was observed in the hospital until another five hours went by and sure enough, his white cell count in his blood began to rise. He was operated on and his inflamed appendix was removed.

This case demonstrates several points.

Just as Sir Zachery described in 1922, an elevated white cell count in the peripheral blood is a *late* sign of appendicitis.

The boy and his family got a $1,000.00 test that was not very helpful in making the diagnosis.

Surgical review committees and insurance companies need to ease up a bit, for if a surgeon doesn't take out a few normal appendixes, the risk of having one perforate by waiting too long increases. The diagnosis was made initially by history and physical exam, the radiological and laboratory tests are only to confirm or deny the diagnosis. And you know, that is the way it is in most of the world of medicine.

In the course of day to day practice, I see patients with smoldering gall bladders, stomach ailments of all kinds, diverticulosis and diverticulitis and myriad types of diarrhea and vomiting. But, when I ask,

"Are you hungry?" and receive a positive reply, I know I can relax, put my feet up and have the luxury of temporizing to sort things out a bit.

On the other hand, when the patient com- plains of no appetite, I know that something is amiss. It may be mild and simple like a stomach virus or something dramatic and life threatening like a perforated ulcer.

Long standing nausea or lack of appetite has an entirely different list of possibilities -- kidney failure, cancers of diverse types, depression, and failure of the cardiopulmonary system.

Hidden infections

Harboring a smoldering infection in the body may cause anorexia and weight loss. They may be difficult to diagnose unless one thinks along those lines.

Hepatitis

Hepatitis is an inflammatory disorder of the liver caused by viruses, chemicals, toxins, and rarely auto-immune reactions. It makes you feel sick. Sometimes it is very sneaky; you can't eat.

Viral hepatitis is caused by one of several hepatitis viruses. We name them A, B, C and I un- derstand there is D, E and F also, yet to be further defined. They are usually transmitted as follows:

Hepatitis A - Fecal oral route - unclean hands, shell-fish from sewage-contaminated areas. There is now a new vaccine for those who are at high risk. I should probably get this vaccine as I love raw oysters and eat them often. HHHmmm...maybe sometime soon.

Hepatitis B - This is the classic, more serious one transmitted by transfusions, intravenous drug abuse, and by accidental needle sticks in a medical setting. The U.S. blood supply is routinely screened for this virus. About one percent of people who get this will have a very bad case -- their livers will be destroyed and they will die. About ten percent will not get over the infection but will develop chronic hepatitis.

EATING

Recently, it was mandated that all Ohio schoolchildren are to be vaccinated for this virus before they can enter school. Perhaps this is a good idea in that some schoolchildren might be tempted to shoot up drugs in the lavatories. Perhaps this is a bad idea in that I doubt in the history of the state, no child ever got hepatitis at school. What I do know is that it was a political idea driven by two groups. The vaccine manufacturers lobbied long and hard to get Ohio legislators to come around to this idea. Millions of dollars were at stake in this bonanza. The second group was the secular humanists and the homosexual lobby working in concert. Their drumbeat is and has been, "We're all at risk...we're all at risk, behavior doesn't matter, morality doesn't matter, we're all at risk."

Hepatitis C - This virus is the new kid on the block but getting a lot of attention. Most of what was called "Non-A. Non-B hepatitis " in years past is hepatitis C. Transmitted by needle stick, blood transfusion, tattoos, and sexual exposure, this virus will slowly destroy the liver over a period of years.

Tuberculosis

The old white plague is still with us, and becoming more resistant to medicines. Again, unless the physician has suspicion to think of this illness, he won't do the specific tests necessary to identify the bacteria.

I recall that my uncle always had a limp. I was told he had tuberculosis of the ankle and spent many months in a TB sanitarium and almost had to have an amputation. Nowadays TB of the ankle would be exotica of the first order and I probably wouldn't recognize it if it bit me on the leg (so to speak).

The clinical signs of tuberculosis are weight loss, night sweats and fevers and possibly chronic cough. Unfortunately, new and powerful strains of this bacterium have emerged in the past decade–strains resistant to all antibiotics.

Bacterial Endocarditis

Infection of the heart valves is a very serious disorder. It is very hard to eliminate the infection. When colonies of bacteria take up residence on the heart valves, showers of bacteria are released into the bloodstream causing chills, fevers, sweats, anorexia and weight loss.

With our aging population, we can expect more of these cases as we have more and more people living into old age, with sclerosed, rough and crinkled up heart valves, perfect homes for a wandering bacterium to take up residence.

AIDS

The AIDS virus can lie dormant for a long time before it starts to make a person sick. When it causes fatigue, malaise and anorexia it is called AIDS-related complex or ARC. When one of the unusual infections occurs, indicating the breakdown of the immune system, then the person has full blown AIDS. The wasting and weight loss so characteristic of this disease is a terrible thing.

Drug toxicity

Adverse reactions to prescription drugs can dampen the appetite, even while they are doing good in other areas, and even when they are in the normal ranges in the blood. Some are quite noted for doing this-

Digitalis

This common heart stimulant and regulator has a narrow therapeutic window -- the difference between a useful dose and a toxic one is very small. It is famous for causing nausea when its levels in the blood creep too high.

Theophyllin

An older medicine for asthma, it has now become a third or fourth line drug for asthma control.

Dilantin

A useful medication for the control of seizures. It sure will make you sick if it goes too high.

EATING

Calcium channel blockers - These very useful blood pressure and angina medicines some- times slow the action of the intestines enough to cause severe constipation. Then the appetite goes down the drain.

Amiodarone (Cordarone) - A newer and useful anti- arrhythmic to control the heart rhythm. Very potent, very useful, and often quite sickening, even in usual therapeutic dosages. Important to find the minimal dosage necessary to control the heart rhythm.

Arthritis medicines - All arthritis medicines can cause stomach upset and all arthritis medicines can cause the stomach to bleed. It doesn't matter if they are the older naproxen or the newer COX II inhibitors. They all have the capacity to upset the equilibrium of the stomach.

Environmental toxins

This is an unusual cause of sickness and anorexia but it does happen.

I recall one young man who came to me for fatigue and weight loss. His hands were quite dirty with grime embedded under the fingernails. I asked him what he did for a living and he said he worked in a salvage yard cleaning auto parts. I asked him if he used any solvents. He said his usual job was to dip parts into tri-cloroethylene to de-grease them, **with no gloves on.** I knew what his laboratory values would be before I ordered them. I told him, "You are destroying your liver with that solvent," and sure enough when his lab values came back, his liver enzymes were ten times normal. Fortunately, he was young and vigorous and by staying away from the offending poison and changing his work habits he recovered completely in short order.

To summarize - *if your appetite is poor, there is something wrong with you.* If weight is dropping off in an unexplained fashion, you are probably sick, so go to the doctor. It's probably not all in your head - it's probably in your heart, lungs, stomach, bowels or liver!

4
Moving....

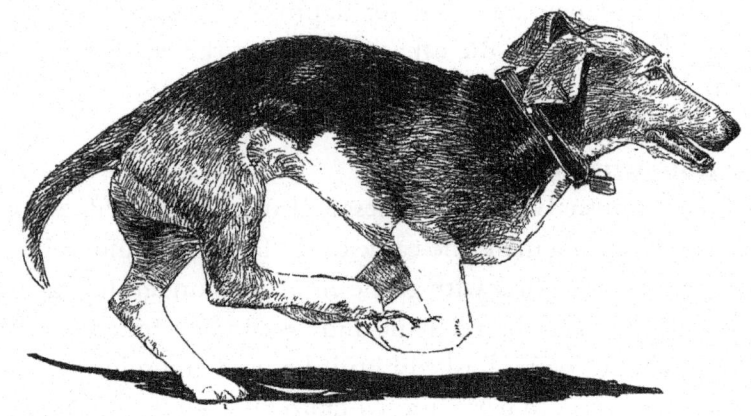

    Moonlight filtered through the branches as I looked up, lying on my back.
    "What a lovely night" I thought. I had fallen down a bank and was staring up at the stars
    I heard a chainsaw of a voice cut through the evening stillness
    "That dog is getting pretty far ahead, we'd best hurry on."
    At least I wasn't lost any more!
    Junior Quillen adjusted his headlight and gave it a shake, "sometimes this silly thing goes out on me."
    "You don't think that dog is running deer, do you?" I offered, climbing to my feet. No raccoons had been detected in several hundred bramble-choked yards.

"That no good so-and-so (not exact quote) better not be running deer!"

"Which direction do you hear him?" Junior asked, pulling out one of his hearing aids and tapping it against a tree.

I strained to hear the dog against the rustling of the wind in the leaves.

The distant barking of the dog changed to a short staccato "chop."

"He's treed one!" Junior shouted. We both set off like madmen up the hill.

The ability to move around as you wish, to walk as far as you'd like for as long as you'd like--these are wonderful gifts. Unfortunately, for many people, they slip away due to neglect, disease, and disuse. Movement and life go hand and hand.

Obesity -The American Plague

It is now official. Over 50% of Americans are overweight. A simple majority. No other demographic group is as large. The implications of this situation are truly staggering both physiologically and financially.

Thousands of books and articles of every description have been written on the subject of obesity. Many scientific journals are devoted exclusively to research on it. Americans spend 33 billion dollars a year on diet aids, clubs, supplements, and exercise equipment; a figure which exceeds the GDP of over one hundred countries. In spite of all these efforts and expenditures, the problem has gotten very much worse over the past two decades.

The economic costs of obesity are enormous. Wolf and Colditz estimate the toll annually as follows:
Direct Cost:$32.4billion
Indirect cost:$30.74 billion

These numbers are so astronomical because obesity affects nearly every organ system of the body, aggravating high blood pressure, arthritis, diabetes and its vascular complications (coronary artery disease, kidney disease and blindness), and several cancers such as colon cancer, prostate cancer, breast cancer and ovarian cancer.

These numbers are truly staggering in import. Yet our population has no incentive rally to change. Our health care system is designed to provide unlimited services to any eligible Medicare patient regardless of wealth or self-inducement of their disorder. The ability of most bypass surgeries to succeed has created complacency in the populace. Why diet or maintain health? One can just get a bypass later when Medicare will cover it. Same thing applies with hip and knee replacements. They are done so routinely on anyone now that there isn't even any discussion on why this came about or if any lifestyle modification should be done to prevent the next one.

There are other sweeping societal changes that contribute to our obesity. In 1965 Americans spent 600 million dollars on fast food. In 1999 we spent 60 billion -- an increase by a factor of one hundred in three decades. That represents a tremendous change in eating habits, leaning toward a much higher fat diet.

Many children now find themselves in communities where it is not safe to play outdoors. This and the burgeoning video game industry have changed the play habits of youngsters throughout the U.S.

The (BMI) is a calculation that can be used to measure both overweight and obesity in adults. It is the measurement of choice for many obesity researchers and other health professionals. BMI is a direct calculation based on height and weight, and it is not gender-specific. Most health organizations and published information on overweight and its associated risk factors use BMI to measure and define overweight and obesity. BMI does not directly measure percent of body fat, but it provides a more accurate measure of overweight and obesity than relying on weight alone.

BMI is found by dividing a person's weight in kilograms by height in meters squared.

The mathematical formula is: weight (kg)/height squared (m2).

To determine BMI using pounds and inches, multiply your weight in pounds by 704.5, then divide the result by your height in inches a second time. I have provided a simplified table to allow you to see where you fall.

This table is accurate 99 percent of the time, in that only rarely do I come across a body builder who is so muscular that they calculate out to be obese. For the rest of us, it is a very good guide.

A BMI over 25 suggests overweight, while a BMI over 30 means you are obese.

Homeostasis

"The process of staying the same." This term was coined in 1930 by physiologist, Walter Cannon. The body has many mechanisms in play to keep the levels of activities the same. Some of these functions under homeostatic control include blood pressure, kidney function, temperature, and oxygen content of the blood.

Unfortunately for dieters, the homeostatic mechanism of the body works to keep the body at the same weight as before, slowing down the breaking down of fat. The dieting body perceives itself as starving. This powerful mechanism is what usually defeats dieters as their weight loss slows and stalls out.

Exercise usually overrides this mechanism to continue the weight loss. I remember vividly when I was in medical school, I took up running. I got into a routine that I would run two to three miles every other day. My weight dropped dramatically even though I was eating anything and everything I could. Form follows function, and the body has a remarkable ability to remodel and change itself if we give it a chance.

I have interviewed and treated all sorts of dieters, of whom 90 percent will fail and return to their pre-dieting weight because of lack of exercise. The conversation goes something like this. . .

Me - "Now, what kind of new exercise program are you going to start doing along with your new diet?"

Patient - "Oh, I get plenty of exercise at work."

Me - "You mean you have a new job?"

Patient - "Oh no, I've had the same job for ten years."

Me - "Well, obviously that's hardly enough, because you are still sixty pounds overweight.

In the over-forty age group, I've identified very few people who have hobbies any more. A few bowlers here and there, no bird watchers, no painters, no hikers, no canoe people, just a lot of going out to eat and watching TV. People who have constructive hobbies are a lot thinner than those that don't. People who are passionate about their hobbies sometimes forget to eat.

Beginning to exercise

The journey of a thousand miles begins with a single step.
-*Chinese proverb*

Many people have the misconception that it takes a grand program or fancy equipment to exercise -- it does not at all. You will advance in stamina and flexibility by starting to do simple exercise right in your living room.

Exercise is even more important for the elderly than it is for the young! The ability to retain one's capacity and function in late middle age and older is dependent on keeping active and exercising. The body never loses its ability to respond nor benefit from exercise, no matter how old the person.

Every person should have a checkup with their physician before starting a new exercise program!

Hypothyroidism "cold and slow"

I most often encounter this disorder in patients who want to lose weight and cannot. It's extremely frustrating for them, but sometimes it really is a glandular condition that is keeping them from losing their extra pounds.

The thyroid gland is a delicate organ, which controls the rate of metabolism of the body. The rate of fat burning and consumption of energy is regulated by the thyroid. If it is malfunctioning, the person will find it nearly impossible to lose weight.

I have treated obesity with medications for some time, recognizing the great threat it poses to health. I have felt for a long time it is well worthwhile to pull out all the stops when it comes to this condition, given the ravages of obesity on the body with time.

I have noticed many times, that even if a patient is given a calorie burning medicine such as phentermine, the patient will not lose weight if they suffer from hidden hypothyroidism. When the missing thyroid hormone is replaced, then the exercise and diet regimen can take hold and the weight will drop off.

Thyroid hormone (and its lack) affects every organ system in the body. The person lacking in thyroid hormone may suffer from a wide variety of complaints and disorders. They include:

- Constipation
- Swelling of the extremities
- Sleep disturbances

- Fatigue
- Dry skin and hair
- Elevated cholesterol
- Mental dullness and even dementia
- Inability to lose weight

I have recently been aggressive in checking thyroid levels in every pre-menopausal woman who turns up with high cholesterol. About a third have sub-clinical hypothyroidism!

The case of Lori B.

A young woman came to me suffering from depression, fatigue and bipolar illness. She was on two antidepressants and large doses of the atypical antipsychotic drug Geodon.

I checked her thyroid numbers and her TSH was mildly elevated (in the 4-5) range and her t3 was low. I started her on levothyroxin and later Armour thyroid because she did not convert t4 to t3 well. The addition of thyroid hormone cured her. Her mind and mood improved dramatically and within a year she was off all psychiatric medicine.

In years past, one could tour any state mental facility and pick out at least one psychotic patient who was suffering from terminal hypothyroidism (myxedema madness) just from their facial appearance. Hypothyroidism can be subtle and insidious as can be!

Recent studies show that up to ten percent of people over 65 suffer from a degree of hypothyroidism! Often the symptoms are subtle and not easy to spot. It is well worth checking a serum TSH level in a person with mild depression, fatigue or forgetfulness.

"Doc. I'm short-winded"

Restriction in the ability to walk is often due to problems of the heart and lungs. Sometimes they are quite subtle and hard to sort out... most are not however.

Heart disease

When the pump that circulates the oxygen carrying blood to the body malfunctions, the ability to walk briskly degrades rapidly. This usually takes the form of three distinct types.

Coronary artery disease

This is the most common form of heart disease in the U.S. today. The coronary arteries supply oxygen rich blood to the heart muscle. When these arteries become plugged with cholesterol, sometimes a sickening pain, an intense squeezing is felt, often running down the arms. That is the classic case, and any third year medical student could diagnose it. Unfortunately, the first manifestation of coronary disease in one third of cases is sudden death!

Now I don't really believe this. Very likely these people had some telltale signs before their hearts went into a deadly irregular rhythm. A subtle squeeze when walking or climbing stairs, some odd indigestion after a heavy meal or just being out of breath frequently could signal coronary artery disease. Sometimes the only symptom is a subtle heaviness or inability to climb stairs or walk as briskly as before.

Too often, these symptoms occur in bull headed men who pride themselves in not going to doctors and being tough guys. They minimize the severity and seriousness of their symptoms, and too often they drop over from a deadly arrhythmia...not really "sudden death."

The risk factors for developing coronary heart disease are well known. Elevated cholesterol, cigarette smoking, a high stress lifestyle, and diabetes all put one at risk, in an additive fashion.

I looked at the man on the exam table and pointed at his chart. "You have gained weight again and your blood sugars are worse than last time!"

J.R. looked sheepish, "Gee Doc, we just finished the holidays, gimme a break."

I noticed the bulge in his shirt pocket and pulled out a pack of Marlboro cigarettes. I looked at his fingernails

"Still a pack a day?"

He grabbed them back, but I wasn't through.

"You have three very bad risk factors for heart disease...diabetes, smoking and high cholesterol. I'll bet you one hundred dollars that you will have a heart attack within five years!"

J.R. looked shocked. "You mean that? That's not very nice. You are supposed to help me."

I stared back with sadness, because without any real psychic ability, I could see the future and it wasn't good.

(J.R. had his heart attack and a three vessel bypass one year and three months later.)

Valvular heart disease

This type of heart disease is really quite simple -- the valves that control the blood flow between the chambers of the heart wear out. These problems are usually congenital or from rheumatic fever as a child. Just like the valves on a car, they always get worse, never get better, and if left too long will ruin the larger structure (the heart).

Serious valvular disease always has murmurs, which are audible with a stethoscope.

A diagnostic test called an echocardiogram can give an accurate picture of the degree of valvular damage and the heart muscle function itself. This is useful in trying to gauge whether the dysfunction of the heart is progressing rapidly.

The trick is to replace the damaged valve, not too early and not too late.

Cardiomyopathy

The subtlest cause of a poorly working heart pump is a sick heart muscle. The most common cause of this is a viral infection that infects the heart muscle, causing a poor contraction of the muscle cells. This can come on quite insidiously and quite frankly, can strike anyone without warning. The victim of such a virus may notice shortness of breath or swelling in the legs as the heart muscle becomes weaker. Many times the heart muscle will get better from this insult and the person can get back to regular activity. Excessive alcohol consumption can poison the heart muscle as well and over time, render it weak and flabby.

Asthma -- on the rise

Many of the major diseases of the adult are decreasing. Heart disease is dropping rapidly due to awareness of the role of blood pressure and cholesterol in the genesis of coronary heart disease. The rate of many cancers is on the decline as well. Not so for asthma. Over the past two decades, we have seen a very significant rise in both adult asthma and childhood asthma as well.

Asthma is an inflammatory condition in which the small bronchial airways constrict due to irritation. During the constriction of the airways, the sufferer feels "tight in the chest," or may even have audible wheezing.

There is a definite subset of asthmatics that wheeze or feel constriction most with exercise. In these people, exercise is their most potent trigger and some may feel little problem at any other time. It is unknown if this is a special type of asthma or just poorly controlled patients who wheeze when they try to run.

In years past, we spoke of "intrinsic asthma" in that the patient "just had it" and no existing stimulus could be found. I no longer believe in intrinsic asthma. I believe all asthma is caused by outside triggers reacting with the body- be they molds, pollens, chemicals, dusts or foods.

It is intriguing to speculate on what is triggering the rise in asthma in our society. Here are a few ideas...

Increased outdoor air pollution

- Probably not -- in that asthma is rising in notorious communities such as Pittsburgh, Pennsylvania and Youngstown, Ohio,

where the quality of air is much improved with the demise of the steel mills. After enactment of the Clean Air Act of 1970, air quality in many other communities is improving as well, yet asthma is increasing.

Increased daycare for young children - The skyrocketing divorce rate and changing work habits of women in the past thirty years has put many young children in daycare settings where early infections such as respiratory syncytial virus is very common. Asthma is more common in children who have had RSV infection in their early infancy. Childhood poverty also causes infants to be exposed to more allergens in their first few months and even before birth. Exposure to dust, mold and cockroach antigens are potent inducers of allergy in the first months of life.

Building techniques - The increased use of formaldehyde-containing particleboard in construction and the burgeoning mobile home population (divorce once again) is a potent stimulus for asthma. The emphasis on energy efficiency and tight houses in recent years increases problems with indoor allergens and molds. Recent trends toward building with synthetic materials and plastic instead of wood and stone seem to stimulate asthma in children.

Low rates of breast feeding - Scientific studies have shown over and over the benefits of breastfeeding on the prevention of allergies and asthma. The Academy of Pediatrics in their latest position paper recommends breast feeding for the first year. Their position paper with over *one hundred* literature references is located on-line at www.aap.org/policy/re9729.

Asthma is a balancing act

The asthmatic can live with low levels of bronchospasm most of the time if they have a sedentary lifestyle. Exertion often is a reliable stimulus to the lungs and they cannot keep up with demand. Thus, the poorly controlled asthmatic starts to wheeze or they just poop out way before they should.

The use of Peak Flow Meters by asthmatics at home has revolutionized asthma therapy. They can avoid severe asthmatic attacks by early intervention.

To re-emphasize -- asthma is an ***inflammatory*** disorder caused by a person reacting to their environment--be it chemicals, foods or dust and molds. Avoidance of the allergens is a foundation for good asthmatic control. If the patient is not willing or able to avoid the allergens exciting their asthma, they will need more layers of medicine to keep them under control. The two are in balance to keep the asthmatic functioning.

Asthmatics need to strive for good control of their disease. Long-term poor control causes changes in the lung similar to that of emphysema over a period of years. With the new medicines available and the knowledge of allergic provocations, most asthmatics can be controlled so their activity is not significantly limited, and they live normal life spans.

Arthritis

I know very little about arthritis, but I will share that little bit with you...some simple facts and some speculations.

Arthritis of the extremities is mostly related to overweight and obesity. No one risk factor is more important than body weight in the development of arthritis of the knees and hips. It is the knees and hips that usually keep people from going and doing, not the feet and ankles in the majority of cases.

Exercise helps arthritis. In most cases, moderate non-impact exercise will help with the stiffness and pain of arthritis. Some authors speculate that movement in the joint is necessary for the cartilage to retain its resiliency. The normal activity of the chondrocytes (cells which make cartilage) depends on stimulation. Thus, inactivity actually causes the cartilage to "wither away."

I know one woman who took up a program of swimming to ease the pain of her arthritis. After some months, she had discontinued all of her pain and arthritis medicines and was quite pain free, due to her exercise program. Swimming, being a non-weight bearing exercise, is the activity par excellence for arthritis in that it is a great workout without any pounding of the joints. Exercise helps until the cartilage is badly worn away, then the grinding of "bone to bone" is no longer helped by additional activity.

Diet may be related to the development of arthritis. Recent studies show strong correlation with the levels of carotenes such as lutein and betacryptoxanthin (found in spinach, collard, kale and broccoli) in resisting the development of osteoarthritis.

Auto-immune diseases

A group of disorders called *auto-immune* diseases are some of the most mysterious, destructive disorders in the realm of medicine. In these problems, patients develop rogue antibodies, which start to attack their own tissues. Some of these disorders include lupus erythematosus, rheumatoid arthritis, polymyalgia rheumatica, systemic sclerosis, Sjogren's syndrome, and a heterogeneous group of disorders known as mixed connective tissue disorder.

No one knows for sure the cause of any of these disorders or why the body should start to attack itself.

A case of Lupus Erythematosus caused by food allergy

K.H. is a 30 year-old female who had suffered from ANA positive (antibodies in her bloodstream) lupus erythematosus for several years. The disorder had affected several of her organ systems including her joints, her heart, muscles and eyes.

At her first visit, she wore dark, wrap-around glasses similar to those worn in years past by cataract patients. Her eyes were so sensitive to light that she wore these huge blinders whenever she was outside of her home. She was on several heart medicines due to heart rhythm irregularities and high blood pressure. She also suffered from joint aches and swelling, skin rashes and migraine headaches.

Skin testing showed her to be allergic to **milk** products, **corn**, **wheat** and **yeast**. She began to eliminate these items from her diet... bread, rolls, pasta, vinegar and all foods containing cornstarch, corn syrup and corn itself.

After a few days, her headache and joint aches began to improve. A little later, her light sensitivity went away and she able to discontinue her dark glasses and her eye drops.

She stayed strictly on her diet and she was able to discontinue her heart medicines and no longer had difficulty walking long distances. After one year, her blood work had returned to normal, her ANA titers (a serum blood test used to gauge the activity of the disease) had returned to normal and she was able to obtain health insurance again!

This most dramatic case shows that the combination of food fragments and her own antibodies caused inflammation in a wide variety of organ systems. Her heart, blood vessels, eyes and joints all were under assault from rogue antibodies depositing in her tissues.

There have been several intriguing studies published regarding arthritis and food reactions.

Panush et al. describe a case of a woman who developed full blown acute arthritis each time she drank milk. Her joints would become hot and red and her blood sedimentation rate would skyrocket with each exposure. This would happen even though she was administered the offending substance in a blinded fashion. Dr Panush then did a study to try and find out how frequent this type of phenomenon actually happened. He fasted a group of patients who had rheumatoid arthritis and then re-introduced foods to see how many of these arthritis patients reacted to food stuffs. Only five percent could be demonstrated to have reproducible reactions to food that caused arthritis. After the study, a couple of the patients stayed on their diet because they had received so much benefit. A 2001 study from Sweden showed 40% of patients with rheumatoid arthritis responded to eliminating grains (gluten) and milk. There is so much anecdotal evidence from patients for this, that researchers keep coming back to the intriguing question "Does diet affect arthritis?"

Richard Feynman the Nobel laureate once said "It is important not to fool yourself, because *you* are the easiest person to fool." This is a point well taken because to assume that all auto-immune diseases are caused by allergies is a mistake. In my practice, the percentage is perhaps a bit higher than that obtained by Dr. Panush but I have a self-selected population. The ones that might respond are those patients who also have problems such as migraine, chronic sinus problems, colitis, eczema and more traditional allergies such as hay fever.

Many patients who come to me have *already* experimented with their diets for some time and perhaps have had a degree of success. These have already suspected what their problem is and just need a little clarification. Some patients have significant chemical sensitivities and their auto-immune problems come from that quarter. These could come from workplace, home, or hobbies. At present, I don't go to people's homes to do detective work, but really, that would make perfect sense, and I am going to start soon. I'll snoop around looking for volatile smells, leaky roofs (mold), and backyard toxic waste.

Many patients have a point of no return. Their immune systems are so sick that the rogue antibodies have no control or inhibition whatsoever and even strict environmental control will not reverse the process and cause improvement or cure. This is sad, because I know several patients who have crossed from the realm of the allergic to the world of auto-immune diseases just because they were too busy to clean up their environmental reactants.

Norman Cousins, in his dramatic book <u>Anatomy of an Illness</u>, relates how after he spent a particularly stressful trip to Moscow he developed ankylosing spondylitis, a painful rheumatoid condition involving pain, inflammation and stiffening of the spine. He tells how he was sleep deprived (no, he wasn't worked over by the KGB, he just had a very taxing schedule) and constantly exposed to diesel fumes in his hotel room. This makes perfect sense to me and there is evidence in the literature to support this view of toxic genesis of auto-immune disease.

Mr. Cousins cured himself from his disorder by a determined program of intravenous vitamin C infusions and laughter. Yes! He had a serious program of watching funny movies several times a day. As he did this, his blood work showed a definite drop in inflammation, week by week of his program.

MOVING....

Use it or lose it

Ages ago Hippocrates stated, "that which is used develops, that which is not used wastes away."

I have noticed over thirty years of clinical practice that this is very true. A sedentary lifestyle is the greatest enemy to health there is. I recently reviewed all my patients with hip and knee replacements and the vast majority were obese. Conversely, I have several patients who have worked at hard physical labor all their lives and are vigorous and still working even in their eighties. Hard work not only never killed anyone but it seems to be very protective!

The situation is even more dire than this. Many studies now coming out suggest that a sedentary lifestyle promotes mental decline as well as physical decline. Two large scale research studies have followed elderly persons over several years measuring the rate of decline of mental ability. The differences were great between the two groups - brisk walking was very protective against loss of mental functioning. It would appear a brisk one-mile walk, taken every other day will do very much for health. Starting in your forties, continue into your fifties, sixties, seventies, eighties and nineties. Why quit? It's rather good for you.

Do Your Bowels Work Freely And Regularly Without The Need of Laxatives?

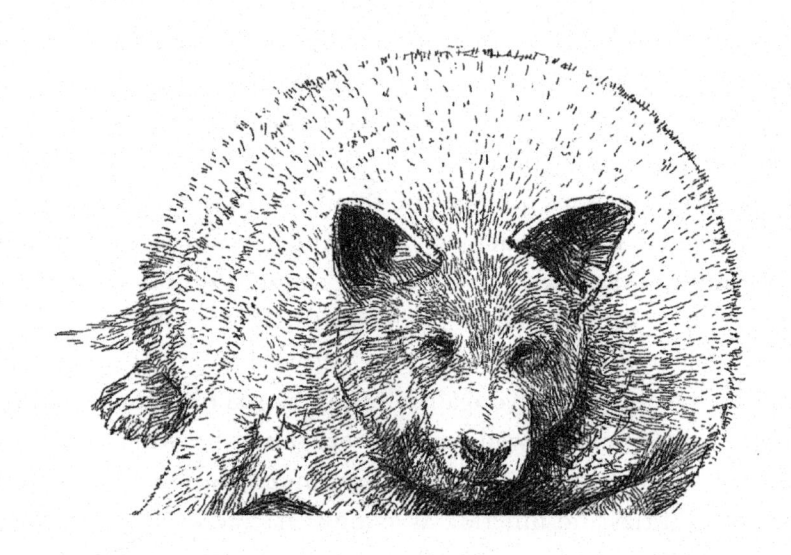

I peered over the black lab table and into the pan. There lay two kidneys, a heart, a spleen, a liver, and part of a colon. Across the table sat a plump, jolly man who was picking the last bits of his lunch from his beard.

"Now, ladies and gentlemen, who can tell me what is wrong with that colon."

Dr. Davies was always so patient, for as first year medical students we were so afraid to venture a guess, we...were...numbskulls actually.

"It has holes in it! Yes, holes! And what do you suppose those holes are called?" (He picked a bit of candy from his pocket and poppedit into his mouth).

"Diverticuli! Quite right, quite right, lads!"

The flower of the British Empire had landed at Albany Medical College during the 1970s and we were the undeserving heirs to didactic methods abandoned almost everywhere else in the twentieth century. The luminaries included Dr. Davies from Uganda, Dr. Scott from Canada and most flamboyant of all was Dr. Oram who trekked and fought with Lord Mountbatten in Burma.

Dr. Davies cleared his throat and disturbed my daydreams of Kipling and Empire…

"Americans are the most constipated people on earth."

At times, he would also intone solemnly..

"In Africa, the chronic diseases of the bowel, that is, cancer and diverticulosis, are virtually unknown." Sometimes he would say both, but a medical student quickly got the idea that bowel disorders were related to diet!

I have thought about what he said many times throughout the years, asking myself, "How can it be that the people in one culture are so ridden with bowel problems and the people of another are so trouble free?" I believe the answer lies in the diet, totally. The function of the bowels is a sensitive indicator of general health and well-being. When they are not working right, then the rest of you probably has some difficulty as well.

I maintain that for proper health, everyone should move their bowels at least daily. With an optimum diet, more than once a day is probably more healthful.

Let's examine what the bowels really do. When stool is passed from the small bowel to the colon, it is liquid, but all the nutrients have been removed. The remaining task is to extract water from the mass (conserving water is a valuable thing!) and to store the remaining bulk until a convenient time to expel it. The stool contains fibrous material of fruits and vegetables, which were not able to be absorbed in the small intestine. It also contains poisons that the liver has detoxified and expelled in the stool.

The detoxifying function of the liver is extremely important. Every strange chemical we ingest such as car exhaust, lacquers, thinners, paint fumes, lead and formaldehyde that out-gases from construction materials all have to be converted to forms that can be excreted, and are expelled in the stool. The liver takes these toxins and combines them with other benign molecules (gluconate mostly) and then excretes them in the bile. The point is, it is not very healthy to have this type of material sitting against the wall of the colon too long...it causes cancer!

A case in point is the family barbecue grill. Frying a nice juicy steak allows juices to drip downward onto the coals and then the smoke rises back up onto the meat. This process cycles over and over until one has some pretty exotic molecules coating your sirloin. These are cancer producing. Recent studies show that grilling more than twice a week increases the rate of colon cancer and even more so if you eat the meat well done.

The Food Pyramid -A Possible Ideal?

A few years ago, the U.S. Dept. of Agriculture came out with the food pyramid - a sort of eating guide for Americans. I consider this guide one of the best things our government has done in the past fifty years. It provides excellent advice on healthy eating.

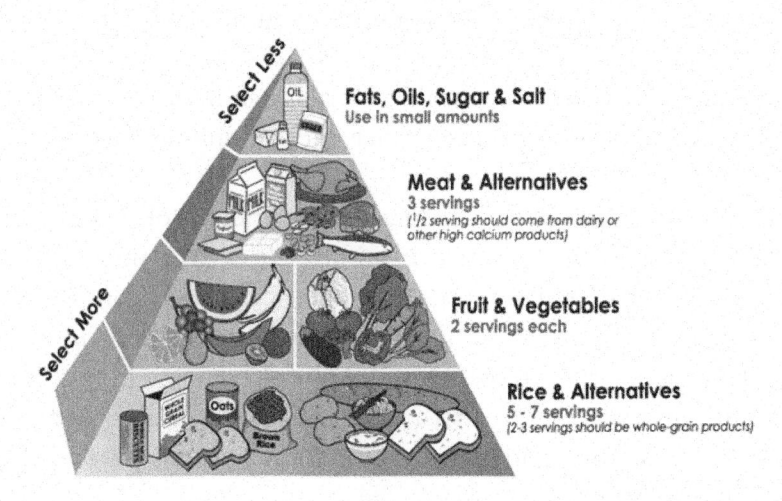

The second tier of this scheme recommends 2-4 fruits per day, PLUS 3-5 vegetables servings a day! Most Americans don't nearly reach that level and don't worry about it either. (Ignorance is bliss in this case, and also terminal constipation!) Following these recommendations

ELIMINATION

would provide a very healthy amount of dietary fiber and go a long way toward eliminating constipation, high cholesterol, so called "spastic colon" disorder, and the worst disorder of all, colon cancer. Actually, this is a vast understatement. If everyone followed these dietary recommendations, nearly every doctor in the country would have to find other employment!

Americans are overfed and undernourished and do not receive enough vitamin C, carotenoids and antioxidants. The government recently raised the recommendation level of vitamin C from 50 mg a day to 90 mg. This is definitely a step in the right direction. The previous level was not one to promote health, but merely enough to keep your teeth from falling out from scurvy. Other recommended daily allowances (RDAs) are being re-examined as well, updated from the 19th century concepts of preventing diseases to those of maintaining optimal health.

The typical American diet contains large amounts of fat, protein, and refined sugars and starches. Grains and fruits are processed to the point where they contain calories, but no vitamins, minerals or fiber.

An improved sample diet might go as follows:

Breakfast a bowl of whole grain cereal with slices of apple or peaches or blueberries on top (one fruit)

Mid-morning snack - small bunch of grapes and a few nuts (one fruit)

Lunch salad with egg or chicken, tomato slices and pears (one fruit, two vegetables)

Supper pizza with peppers, mushrooms and pineapple (two vegetables, one more fruit)

Let's try a different day, with other combinations:

Breakfast leftover pork-chop microwaved and a bunch of grapes. (I have long considered the combination of the hot and greasy meat and the cold and juicy fruit an excellent and interesting contrast)

<u>Mid-morning snack</u> - hand full of walnuts

<u>Lunch</u> grilled cheese sandwich and small salad (no fries please!) with sliced fruit

<u>Supper</u> sirloin steak, steamed broccoli with butter, tomato slices with vinaigrette, and fruit salad
I count three fruits and three vegetables for this day.
This is the type of diet that will provide the adequate amounts of antioxidants that will keep the body well.

Antioxidants - What They Are, Why We Need Them

In addition to the basic vitamins and minerals, there is an additional class of nutrients receiving much attention recently ...the antioxidants. These are chemicals that prevent damage to our cell membranes and DNA. To put it quite simply, we *rust*! Oxidation of our cells occurs especially from very active oxygen molecules such as super oxides. These are various compounds containing one or more oxygen atoms, which have donated an electron in a chemical reaction. These oxygen species are very reactive, and can damage neighboring proteins comprising the cell membranes of organs and even the very DNA itself.

Some of the important antioxidants are familiar to all of us. Vitamin C is an antioxidant and so is beta-carotene. There are many others that are not so familiar but which are potent protectors just the same.

Here is a list of some of the protective champions that should be in everyone's diet:
<u>Lycopene</u> found in tomatoes and red berries.
<u>Alpha-carotene</u> dark green vegetables and yellow and orange ones. The more potent sister to beta- carotene!

ELIMINATION

<u>Alliums</u> Onions, garlic and leeks all have this potent cell protector

<u>Lutein</u> This antioxidant is getting media attention for its possible role in prevention of macular degeneration.

<u>Zeaxanthin</u> Dark green leafy vegetables like spinach, collards, kale, and chard.

<u>Anthocyanins</u> The blue compounds in blueberries and blackberries- very potent protectors.

Antioxidants protect us from the environmental toxins, which attack our bodies by binding the oxygen products of degradation of pollutants.

Vitamin Supplements - What To Do?

It is much better to obtain the requisite vitamins from fruits and vegetable than by taking vitamins. Vitamins supplements when taken, must be balanced and in appropriate amounts to ensure no harm is being done.

A recent study of men with lung cancer was done to see if supplements with beta-carotene would affect the progression of their tumors. The group with the beta-carotene actually did worse than those with no vitamin supplement at all. Another study shows that supplementation with large doses of beta-carotene actually promotes skin cancer as well.

I feel there is enough scientific data regarding this vitamin to use it with caution. I take a balanced vitamin with several carotenes in it including alpha carotene, lutein, and xanthine, a couple times a week when I feel I haven't eaten enough yellow and bright green vegetables. Several points are worth repeating here...

Large doses of beta-carotene are toxic. I often see vitamins advertised with as much as 20,000 International Units (IU) in a capsule. This is way too much. I never take more than 5,000 units at a time and then never without its fellow carotenoids.

Vitamin supplements with beta-carotene should also contain the other carotenes. These vitamins work together as a team. It may be that larger doses of beta-carotene inhibit the absorption of its teammates from the bowel or possibly inhibit their proper action on a cellular level. There may be yet unidentified factors in fruits and vegetables which large doses of beta-carotene interfere with, for as much as we don't like to admit it, taking a vitamin pill is not the same as eating fresh fruit produce, not by a long shot.

But I hear often, fruits and vegetables are expensive! Well, yes... good foods that have valuable nutrition are going to cost more than poor foods with little value. That makes perfect sense. I guess one needs to account for the expensive illnesses that are down the road for those foolish enough to skimp on fruits and vegetables.

When the Lord made our world and us to live in it, I believe He provided everything we need to eat and live well. Because we are sometimes a little slow (witted), He made things that are especially good for us brightly colored to catch our attention. Thus, if we examine foods high in vitamins and anti-oxidants, it is the deeply and brightly colored ones every time.

Vitamin D - The sunshine vitamin

Vitamin D is routinely tested for and supplemented these days. There is evidence that vitamin D deficiency is related to Multiple sclerosis, and many other diseases. The problem is, oral supplements are absorbed very poorly.

There is scientific evidence that using a tanning booth judiciously in the winter months, tanning the trunk about 5 minutes a week, is twice as effective as taking a high dose of vitamin D

Vitamin D is important in maintaining nerve and brain tissue. Those deficient in Vitamin D are twice as likely to develop Alzheimer's disease. Chronic pain patients will require twice as much narcotic than those with adequate levels of Vitamin D!

The case against fat

"This is a lasting commandment for the generations to come, wherever you live: you must not eat any fat or any blood." Leviticus 3:17

ELIMINATION

This warning, now 6000 years old, was commanded by the Lord for his people, the Israelites. It contains good advice now as then.

Our diet needs a little fat in it, perhaps about 20 to 30 grams a day. We need it because there are three fatty acids that our bodies cannot synthesize by themselves. Those are the "essential fatty acids" i.e. linoleic, linolenic and arachadonic acids. We also need a smidgen of fat to help with the absorption of the fat-soluble vitamins A, D, and E. The American Heart Association recommends a diet that contains no more than 30% fat. For a 2000 calorie diet that turns out to be about 70 grams or two full ounces of fat per day, or the fat in 3/4 of a stick of butter! The fat in a 16-oz (before cooking) sirloin steak amounts to only about 30 grams, so the 30% fat diet is really quite liberal indeed.

In light of the massive obesity and incidence of coronary artery disease in this country, this represents a major challenge. The average American diet contains approximately 40% fat!

The high cholesterol problem is largely driven by dietary fat. Here's how it works...fat, to be absorbed from the small intestine, has to be broken down into small fragments and then bound to bile to be absorbed. Large amounts of fat in the diet ensure that much bile will be manufactured. The body perceives that bile is a valuable commodity, reabsorbing 90% of it from the intestine and sending it back to the liver for reuse. The body re-uses the bile because its large structure required many enzymatic processes to create it. Thus, it was very expensive in terms of energy currency to create.

Bile and cholesterol are only one small biochemical step away from each other, and so when large amounts of bile are produced, a large amount of cholesterol is also . Cholesterol is one of the most versatile compounds in the body in that all the adrenal hormones and all the sex hormones are made directly from it. Unfortunately, the body has no pathways to degrade cholesterol once it is formed.

Fish Oil and Fat

Many studies show beneficial effects from eating fish, particularly cold-water fish such as salmon. Significant decreases in heart disease can be detected by substituting one meal per week from beef and pork to broiled fish. The benefits of fish are attributed to specific oils call Omega-3 free fatty acids.

Cross-cultural studies show that Inuit Eskimos have low rates of coronary artery disease. They do not have a low-fat diet however. Their level of fat intake is nothing short of incredible to maintain their energy in the cold frozen north. Chewing on whale blubber is a favorite treat...not what I'd call low-fat. Most of their fat calories come from the fish of the area particularly salmon, cod, and swordfish, all rich in Omega-3 fatty acids.

Many people take fish oil as a supplement.

Studies show it has some beneficial effects on blood clotting and lowering LDL (bad) cholesterol. It may also lower triglycerides and act as a potent anti-inflammatory to blood vessel walls. However, adding fish oil to an already high-fat diet may actually make serum cholesterol levels worse. What one should do is cut out a couple beef and pork meals a week and replace them with broiled salmon, swordfish, or tuna. Deep fried fish is worse than no fish at all, and doesn't count toward any health benefit whatsoever.

Animal Fats and Cancer

Breast cancer, colon cancer, and prostate cancer are all related to a high-fat diet. The evidence is piling up higher and higher each year, yet most doctors don't advise their patients in diet modification at all.

Many breast cancer studies show that when Japanese women who generally have a low rate of breast cancer immigrate to the U.S., they adopt the cancer rate of their new country. Animal studies show that the Omega-3 fatty acids in fish have a tumor suppressant effect and inhibit the breast cancer cells from developing new blood vessels (angiogenisis).

High levels of antioxidants in the serum of women are a marker for low breast cancer risk. The risk was halved when the rate of the woman with the highest levels were compared with the lowest. Time magazine published a dramatic article with a map called "Breast cancer around the world" This is available online. Go there and click on the various countries….. the difference between the developed countries and undeveloped is amazing!

The case of prostate cancer is even more dramatic. Animal studies show impressive stimulation of tumors in mice fed diets high in saturated fat. Mice fed citrus pulp were protected from the cancer-causing experimental drugs.

Human studies are impressive as well. Men who were scheduled for prostate biopsy were treated for one month only on a very low-fat diet with flax oil supplementation (omega-3s again). When they underwent their biopsies, the aggressiveness of their tumor was significantly different from controls that ate their regular diet.

Another group of men with known prostate cancer were put on very low fat diets with omega-3 fatty acid supplementation. They were followed for several months to track the rise of their PSA (prostate specific antigen) levels. The men on the low-fat diet took over twice as long to double their baseline PSA level -- showing that these supplements had an effect on the aggressiveness of their tumors. Perhaps this is due to the drop of serum testosterone in the low fat group, another observed effect of the diet modification.

Colon Cancer

A diet high in fruits and vegetable has been shown to lower the rate of colon cancer. Dietary studies in many different countries show lower risk in those who consume large amounts of fruits and vegetables and higher risk in those who consume large amounts of animal fat. In fact, the risk seems much more associated with the high animal fat than that with a low fiber diet. The modus operandi in this country is to assume that colon cancer is largely hereditary. We herd up relatives for colon screening if mama is found with a tumor and spend very little time advising dietary changes that will lessen the risk of the same. An underlying problem is that most people don't even know what constipation is! Their minds are so muddled by laxative advertising and by indifferent doctors, that many folks think it's OK to have a bowel movement once a week!

The important elements of healthy bowel function are:

1. Dietary fiber in the form of whole grain cereals, fruits, and vegetables.
2. Adequate water intake to keep the stools moist.
3. Exercise to stimulate the bowels in moving the stool mass along.
4. Opportunity to move the bowels when the urge arises. It is very poor practice to resist the urge to defecate when it arises. Such a habit will cause the stool to get even drier with time and more difficult to pass. It also interferes with the normal muscular action of the lower colon.

The myth of spastic colon disease or irritable bowel syndrome (IBS)

I don't even like to use the term spastic colon, but you've heard it so I guess I have to use it *to debunk* it.

I don't mean to imply that many people's bowels don't work right--that's not true. I read recently on the internet that 40 million persons suffer from irritable bowel syndrome! To imply that 15% of the population has a disorder is quite frightening. Granted, that many people may have trouble with their bowel movements and don't know what to do about it. It would be just as correct to speculate that

15% of the entire population was never taught to eat properly! They have crampy stools and have to run to the bathroom with marked urgency. They have constipation. They can't get their bowels to move no matter what they do.

They have either a poor diet or a poisoned bowel from hidden food allergies.

The Poisoned Bowel

The bowel will not work properly if there are allergic reactions going on inside on a chronic basis. This can take the form of frequent diarrhea, alternate in constipation and diarrhea, and a mostly constipated form. The exact pattern is seen with milk protein allergy in infancy. Some babies will have diarrhea, some constipation, and some will alternate. I believe that these will be some of the very patients that will, thirty years later, be suffering from irregular bowels. Studies involving elimination diets show high percentages of improvement in normalizing bowel function, by identifying and eliminating colonic triggers. Still other studies show many patients improve with the allergic blocking agent cromolyn, further evidence for allergic triggers for at least a large subset of irritable bowel sufferers.

Some new studies show that a very high percentage of spastic colon sufferers have bacterial overgrowth of the small bowel. These patients have improvement with antibiotic treatment. Diagnosis is by breath test to detect the metabolic components of the bacteria. Thus, patients with "irritable bowel syndrome" are really a heterogeneous group still waiting diagnosis.

The Lotronex Debacle

A few years ago, a new drug targeting the urgent diarrhea of spastic colon disorder was removed from the market by the Food and Drug Administration(FDA). This drug had caused several deaths, many hospitalizations, and several colectomies (the colon surgically removed). The drug's manufacturer had published cautions that the drug was not to be used in the constipated variants of spastic colon. The problem with this disorder is that sometimes the patient will have diarrhea, sometime constipation, and sometimes alternation of the two. These things cycle and vary depending on which non-tolerant or allergic foods are being eaten. Thus, it was hard to determine which patient was appropriate for the drug for what time. Use of the drug caused complete shutdown of the bowel when used in the constipated patient. This drug is an off-shoot of another drug used to treat symptoms of migraine (which we will examine shortly). Interestingly enough, I believe that the same errors are being promulgated in that case as well. A drug is being used to treat symptoms and not to treat the basic underlying causes.

An Interesting Case of Colitis

F.B. was a 56-year-old truck driver who was having more and more diarrhea. He was having six to eight bowel movements a day, often with a large degree of urgency. It was interfering with his livelihood.

I inquired into his diet. "Frank, what do you like to eat?"

"Just usual stuff," he replied, "sandwiches. Oh, and lots of milk - five or six glasses a day."

I thought, that can't be healthy – he will start growing ears and a tail.

"That's quite a lot. Why don't you quit for a while?" I offered.

Frank looked puzzled, "I'm not sure I can. I really like it."

Because Frank was having some mucus in his stools, I did a sigmoidoscopy on him and took a few snip biopsies from some areas that were a little inflamed. The biopsy report showed sheets of eosinophils invading the mucosal lining of his colon. These are the classic allergic cells that collect in the noses of hay fever sufferers during ragweed season. Frank had allergic colitis! I finally convinced Frank to lay off the milk completely for a week only. He was surprised when his stools returned to normal almost immediately. I encouraged him to try some frozen yogurt to satisfy his cravings and he found that he could tolerate it well.

This case illustrates a few points that bear repeating:

1. The body will often crave the very thing that is making it sick in order to maintain homeostasis, thus the concept of food addiction is a real one. Children will eat allergic foods nearly to the exclusion of all others. They seem driven in their consumption of the very things making them sick.

2. People will go long periods of time tolerating disease. I guess this comes from not really knowing what is normal and what is not.

3. Frank's colon was visually quite normal, and I could have just as easily decided to not biopsy the areas that were so impressive microscopically. I suspect this happens sometimes when patients have

colonoscopies for irritable bowel syndrome. The visual inspection is important though because a colonic cancer can cause similar symptoms and, of course, one doesn't want to miss those.

4. Although the biopsy was helpful in reinforcing the diagnosis, and convincing the patient of the proper course of action, the diagnosis was really made through history long before any procedure was performed.

The Cave Man Diet

I often recommend that patients go on the simple foods diet or *cave man diet* to see if they can ferret out food reactions that might be responsible for their symptoms. I find that the foods responsible are largely those of civilization. The confections, the candy, and the treats that we eat as staples.

Imagine yourself far away from civilization...your plane has crashed along a stream in Northern Maine. After you build a little shelter from the wind and find a water source, your next concern is food. You recognize several berries that are edible and wolf them down. You start fishing in a nearby stream and catch a nice trout on a piece of yarn and a pin. Digging for roots and gathering acorns you find some starchy food to make a kind of porridge. All these foods are quite different from those comprising your daily diet at home. This type of wild foods diet or wild man diet is used experimentally sometimes to uncover hidden food intolerance.

The diet consists of:

Meats... any you think don't bother you: beef, lamb, woodchuck, rabbit, venison quail, or turkey.

Vegetables... carrots, leeks, brussels sprouts, cabbage, spinach, artichokes, beets...anything really.

Fruits... any and all, unless you think sugars and yeast are a big problem (N.B. I am not a big yeast allergy advocate. I don't deny that some people have chronic problems there, but I just don't think it is nearly the problem that many of its proponents think it is.)

THE WAY OF FIVE

Conversely, the forbidden things are the ones cultivated of civilization:
<u>Wheat and flour items</u> bread, rolls, pizza, cake pie, doughnuts, crackers, hamburger buns.

<u>Corn items</u> corn chips, corn starch, corn syrup (ketchup, barbecue sauce, pancake syrup, most candy, soda pop).

<u>Milk products</u> milk, cheese, yogurt, ice cream, milk chocolate.

<u>Yeast-containing foods</u> vinegar, barbecue sauce, ketchup, salad dressings

<u>Sugar-containing items</u> all the cookies, candy,
cakes, and soft drinks Americans make
the staples of their diets!

After one has lived on meat, vegetables, and fruit for a week, one reintroduces the civilized foods back again, *one at a time* and watches for reactions. In short, this is a gluten-free, lactose-free, and sugar-free diet all in one... that can find food sensitivities very rapidly.

I've presented a potpourri of topics associated with diet and eating, and how foods affect the body and well being. Most of these problems derive from departing from eating *natural* foods and trying to substitute less nutritious, pre-packaged, chemicalized, convenient and often man-made food into the diet.

LE MENTAL.... DER GEIST......................THE MIND...

Are You Cheerful and Productive Every Day?

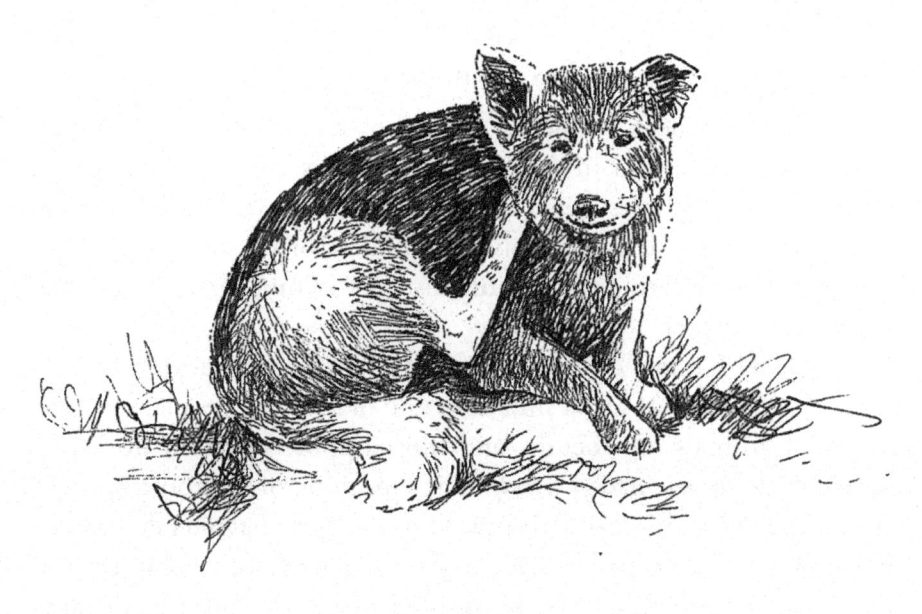

What a piece of work is man!
How noble in reason!
How infinite in faculty!
Hamlet Act ii Sc 2

The working of the human mind is truly something to be viewed with awe.

Shakespeare's words were ironic in that his character, Hamlet, was on the verge of madness and plotting murderous revenge. From the highest peaks of brilliance to the deepest depths of depravity, no other function of any animal is able to span so wide a stream.

Yet the human mind does not always work efficiently. It is prone to psychoses, neuroses, phobias and personality disorders of wide and diverse types. We have a smorgasbord of mental quirks to choose from, and it appears as though everyone gets a little bit of something . Fortunately, in this new millennium, there is greater hope than ever before because of recently discovered interactions between the various body systems, vitamins, environmental toxins, and highly effective medications that are now available.

Anxiety disorders

Anxiety disorders, including agoraphobia, are the most common types of mental illness in America today. This cluster of emotional problems also includes generalized anxiety disorder, post-traumatic stress disorder, social anxiety disorder, and assorted specific phobias. The chance of suffering from **panic** disorder to one degree or another is almost ten percent.

People with panic disorder are fearful. They have fear of traveling, fear of heights, fear of social situations and of meeting people, of closed spaces, of animals, of doctors, and most importantly and ironically, they *fear the panic attack itself.* The emotions of a phobic brought face to face with a bird, or a thunderstorm, or an unavoidable elevator ride approach that of a character of Edgar Allen Poe..... abject terror . No wonder they will go to impossible lengths to avoid experiencing these feelings.

Panic attack symptoms

During a panic attack, some or all of the following symptoms occur:
- Terror- a sense that something unimaginably horrible is about to happen and one is powerless to prevent it
- Racing or pounding heartbeat
- Chest pains
- Dizziness, lightheadedness, nausea
- Difficulty breathing
- Tingling or numbness in the hands
- Flushes or chills

- Sense of unreality
- Fear of losing control, going "crazy", or doing something embarrassing
- Fear of dying

(from National Institute of Mental Health "understanding Panic Disorders")

These sensations often mimic symptoms of a **heart attack** or other life-threatening medical conditions. As a result, the diagnosis of panic disorder is frequently not made until extensive and costly medical procedures fail to provide a physical explanation or provide relief.

Many people with panic disorder develop intense anxiety between episodes. It is not unusual for a person with panic disorder to develop phobias about places or situations where panic attacks have occurred in the past, such as in supermarkets or while traveling. As the frequency of panic attacks increases, these often begin to avoid situations where they fear another attack may occur, or where help would not be immediately available. This avoidance may eventually develop into agoraphobia, an inability to go beyond known and safe surroundings because of intense fear and anxiety.

Panic sufferers describe overwhelming and unpleasant physical sensations during a panic attack, with a great majority reporting shortness of breath or strangulation in extreme cases. Panic disorder patients often present to emergency rooms fearing they are having a heart attack. It is estimated that 16 to 25% of patients presenting in emergency rooms with chest pain have panic disorder. Unfortunately, this problem goes undiagnosed in over ninety percent of the cases!

Agoraphobia: the self made prison

Perhaps you know someone who doesn't go out much, who doesn't enjoy socializing or shopping. They may be suffering from agoraphobia. The name is derived from the Greek roots *agora*, meaning "marketplace", and *phobia*, meaning "fear of."

"Fear of the marketplace" is a very apt term for this condition.

The key element to this disorder is that the person fears leaving their home. Friends and family will notice that the person suffering from agoraphobia will leave the house very little, avoiding most invitations to go shopping or socialize. In interviewing many of these patients, I find that usually there is no distinct place or activity that they fear, but they are in terror of triggering the overwhelming reactions that their body goes through when they panic outside their home. They truly fear ***"fear itself."*** Their hearts start to pound, and it feels as though breathing itself becomes impossible. Indeed, many agoraphobics relate that it is very much like having a heart attack whenever they go shopping! In self-defense, they develop a "safe zone" in which they feel comfortable and then start to avoid going beyond it.

The irony of this condition is that in order to recover from the illness, the sufferer must leave his home and seek treatment. It's like the dilemma of the monkey with his hand caught in the coconut...he can't get unstuck and use his hand again unless he lets go of something he wants very badly. The chimp can always find something else for lunch, but the agoraphobics are so miserable outside their safety zone that letting go of their "coconut" even briefly is more than they are able to do. Many of the more severe sufferers are never able to accomplish this, despite deteriorating health and other problems. They never see the dentist and their teeth become decayed and abscessed. They cannot tolerate going out to see a physician, and so they may develop strange and even disfiguring illnesses, which must become so severe as to be virtually unbearable before they can bring themselves to consult someone. Unfortunately, it is common for them to allow ordinary treatable illnesses to progress beyond the point where medical intervention can help.

Although the media like to print dramatic stories on the housebound agoraphobic, these unfortunates actually represent less than 10% of those that suffer from the problem. Most simply endure the stress and try to function, though they experience much less joy from life than they might. Like walking around with a stone in your shoe, life this way is do-able, but there is too much discomfort for it to be any fun.

The good news is that, like other panic disorders, agoraphobia is very treatable. Anxiety medications and/ or antidepressants are quite effective in providing relief from this illness. Behavioral therapy with a psychologist is also very successful in relieving the panic disorders, with or without medicine. Getting the therapist and patient together is the hard part.

Obsessive-Compulsive Disorder

Doubt
1 a: uncertainty of belief or opinion that often interferes with decision-making
  b: a deliberate suspension of judgment
2 a: state of affairs giving rise to uncertainty, hesitation, or suspense
3 a: a lack of confidence: DISTRUST
  b: an inclination not to believe or accept

Five percent of the United States population suffers from Obsessive Compulsive Disorder to some degree. And rest assured, it is a horrible curse for those who have it, as well as those who live with them. Doubt pervades their lives. Even though they may have checked the house locks ten times before retiring, they still worry whether they have done it correctly, or even if they really checked them at all.

The following case histories illustrate the "doubting disease."
"I would struggle with Obsessive-Compulsive Disorder pretty consistently for the next fifteen years, with most of my obsessions now revolving around the fear of acquiring HIV and AIDS. Although I had no risk factors for getting AIDS, I became absolutely obsessed with the fear of being "contaminated" by the HIV virus. During an 8-year period, I would have more than 40 HIV tests, all negative of course. But due to the doubting nature of ODC, I would no sooner hear a "negative" result from the clinician that I would doubt what I actually heard, doubt the accuracy of the test, doubt the honesty of the doctor

and doubt that the test was even performed. I could think of a million scenarios of why my negative test could not possibly be accurate."

And so it goes with OCD. " It's a never ending circle of doubt and deception. On the very off-chance that I received my "negative" test results on a rather good OCD day for me, I would then walk to my car, perhaps see a Band-Aid lying on the ground and somehow "convince" myself that I now acquired HIV from the Band-Aid. A reason for another test!"

The above case would fall into the category of a person with health related compulsions, in this case, the need to constantly check to see if they had AIDS. Not all persons suffer from the "doubting" form of the disease. In another type, *intrusive and recurring thoughts* will plague the person.

Consider the following case history from the web site "healthy place"

"I was thinking about how we always said we loved God in Sunday school. All of a sudden a thought popped into my head, like a little voice daring me to say the words "I hate God." So I thought the words in my head, "I hate God." I immediately became anxious because I knew that I didn't hate God, the words had just popped into my head without my control. I tried to just shake it off, but the words just kept coming: "I hate God." "I hate God." I started to get really anxious as I was thinking, "Stop it! Why am I saying that? I love God." So I forced myself to say in my head "No, I love God," but it didn't help. The words just kept coming and coming and coming, "I hate God. I hate God." I was fighting back the tears because I was really scared that God could hear me. When I got to school, I was really shaken from what had happened. I tried to forget it, but for the rest of the day it was stuck like a splinter in the corner of my mind. When I got home, I ran to my mother and tried to explain to her what had happened. I was in tears, I was so upset. I tried to explain to her that I couldn't stop saying "I hate God" and was trying to counteract it by saying "I love God." I can still see the perplexed look on her face as she regarded me. I could tell that she knew I was in pain but had no idea why. She told me that it was OK and that I shouldn't worry about it. She comforted me by saying, "I know you love God, it's okay." Even though I was only six years old, I had a feeling that I was being placated (obviously not in a way I could articulate then, but in retrospect, I think I knew). That's where my self-esteem took a downturn, as I became increasingly aware of how different I was.

I wasn't diagnosed with OCD until 16 years later in my senior year in high school. I'd like to think that if I'd been diagnosed earlier, those 16 years in between wouldn't have been fraught with such agony."

Another variant is an obsession with contamination, cleaning, germs or the constant need to wash one's hands. Many OCD sufferers have compulsions to wash their hands in order to constantly rid themselves of germs. The performance of these rituals often consume much of a day.

Many OCD sufferers exhibit magical thinking in their disorder. This is the belief that performing certain actions will cause or prevent events in their lives that have no connection to those actions. I have encountered a patient who felt he had to line up the silverware on the table in just a precise fashion or terrible things would happen to him. Perhaps the old playground chant "step on a crack, break your mother's back" originally came from an OCD sufferer...

Because of OCD, Bill was constantly late.... Getting up took all morning. Brushing his teeth took over an hour. When brushing his hair, he brushed ten sets of ten strokes each. If interrupted or distracted, he had to start all over again... He once went to a restaurant to meet a date for dinner. He went early to freshen up a bit in the bathroom. Unfortunately, he became enmeshed in his rituals. He was surprised when he emerged at 2:00 A.M. and his date wasn't waiting for him!

Some OCD sufferers have superstitious compulsions. One gentleman refused to say the word cat. One woman counted every word so that any sentence would not have thirteen words. Another man tapped each cigarette four times before he would smoke it. One poor woman memorized the classified advertisements in the paper every weekend thinking this would prevent her family from being in a traffic accident. No sufferer has all these components of course, but they are given as examples of the ways in which compulsions can take control of a person's life.

The ugly man syndrome

I have identified several patients who seem to criticize their spouses and children unendingly. Often they are obsessed with tidiness about the home, and it is very important that it be kept completely in order. They seem to live in an unending state of irritability, yelling and snapping all the time, generally "acting ugly." These people seem to be suffering from a variant of OCD with a healthy dose of narcissism!

The whole family is involved…Oh yes! They are. The importance of the rituals cannot be overemphasized. If a spouse or child interrupts the repetition or the counting or the arranging, they will be snapped at, and made to feel unimportant or stupid… so the obsessive can return the mysterious cycles spinning in their brains. The problem of Obsessive Compulsive Disorder frequently seems shameful to the sufferer, and the denial level is high. Often they are reluctant to seek help because their problems seem so odd. I have seen such badly wasted lives and damaged children due to this disease.

There is excellent treatment for this disorder now! The modern drugs called SSRIs often have an immediate and dramatic effect on the course of OCD in 75 percent of cases. Prozac and its newer sisters, Zoloft and Paxil, are all excellent medications. Still not everyone responds equally to medications. So pills are not always "magic bullets" for this disorder. Seeing a psychiatrist or psychologist skilled in behavior therapy is very important for help in interrupting the obsessive's patterns of the past, and giving the sufferer skills to modify and control the behaviors.

Depression

One third of all Americans will suffer from depression during their lifetime. Additionally, it is estimated that up to 5% of persons visiting a family doctor are depressed on any given day! That is certainly a lot of sadness and suffering! Significant depression, called clinical depression, is marked by a withdrawal from life, continuing sadness over a prolonged period of time (months), and the feeling that life is not worth living anymore.

There are several symptoms that are experienced by most depressed people, and they are remarkably similar from one person to the next.

Sadness or depressed mood 89%

Loss of interest or pleasure in activities 80%

Significant weight loss or loss of appetite 65%

Insomnia or hypersomnia (excessive sleep) 60%

Psychomotor retardation or agitation (the sufferer acts lethargic and weary, or nervous and hyperactive) 55%

Loss of energy 50%

Feeling of worthlessness or guilt 45%

Decreased ability to concentrate 40%

Recurrent thoughts of death or suicide 40%

The following case history exhibits many of the features of the depressed episode.

Trapped like a rat

L.S. was a man who hated his job. He had a mid-level manager's job in a large firm with a new boss whom he despised. He was trapped. The children were doing well in school and he felt he couldn't move to another town. His family was well, but they depended on his job for their health insurance. And so he felt that he had no choice but to "tough it out."

He began to lose interest in his work and dreaded getting up in the morning. Sleeping became difficult and he began to awake at 3:00 A.M. every morning. He would walk the halls, toss and turn in bed with sleep eluding him. He often would fall asleep around 5:00 A.M. and when his alarm sounded at 6:30 he felt so terrible he didn't know what to do. (Morning dysphoria) He lost interest in his hobbies. He withdrew from his friends and his sex drive dropped to zero.

L.S. sought help, and was put on an antidepressant. I instructed him to make a list of small but concrete steps he could take to improve his life, make it more enjoyable, and allow him hope for a better future. His list looked like this...

1. Get 15 minutes of exercise a day.
2. Update resume and send it to a job fair
3. Go out with his wife for dinner weekly

L.S. improved rapidly. He had a constructive talk with his boss and was assigned to a new project in which he could utilize his skills more effectively. As he began to realize that he could control greater portions of his life, he began to see hope in the future for himself and his family.

Animal models perhaps demonstrate the way that emotional damage occurs in depressive disorders. Mice and rats that are forced to run a maze continue to do so even if the challenge is made more and more difficult. They will persist even if electrical shocks are applied for wrong decisions, if they can eventually reach the end and get the cheese. If the maze is made impossible, however, the animal will lie down and give up, so much like depressed persons who cannot see any way to improve their situation.

Depression is a deadly disorder. Suicide is the lethal end of one in twenty of these sad people, and even this figure is probably greatly underreported. How many car accidents on dark and rainy nights, or incidents of experienced pilots whose small plane crashed unexpectedly are really an end for depressed people who didn't feel there was any solution to their problem? How many destructive behaviors such as substance abuse, drunk driving, and eating disorders are really suicide on the installment plan?

Medical treatment for clinical depression has been revolutionized with the introduction of new, more effective medications--nearly a dozen in the past ten years. Most depressed people will respond to at least one of the modern antidepressants that we have available. New discoveries about the biochemistry of the brain make it clear that depression is often a chemical imbalance, rather than a character flaw such as "feeling sorry for yourself." As the stigma of depression becomes less and less with the passing of the years, it is devoutly to be hoped that more people will seek treatment and escape from their dark prisons of suffering.

Bipolar disorder (manic -depressive illness)

This disorder is one of the most fascinating of the various mental illnesses. The unique symptom for manic-depressive patients is their tendency to swing between deep-depression and wild euphoria. They can be "down in the dumps" one day and "flying high" the next.

R.J. was a fifty-year-old businessman, a district manager in a large national firm . He had risen through his company rapidly, often putting in long hours. He has long been recognized as an aggressive competitor, often bringing new and exciting ideas to the company.

R.J.'s co-workers noticed that he was becoming more and more irritable, less tolerant of those not "flying with the eagles" as he put it. He began working even longer hours, often well into the night, on "new secret projects." One morning he did not report to work and missed an important meeting. His wife was called and a search was begun. He was found standing on a busy street near his office building. He had draped twenty or more of his neckties around his neck and was holding several aloft, shouting to passing motorists that he was selling his neckties.

In the psychiatric hospital, he was loud and aggressive. He talked rapidly, often speaking familiarly to patients and staff alike. He was intrusive into others' affairs and was nearly assaulted by another patient. R.J. presented elaborately drawn diagrams to his physicians outlining his proper treatment, often embellished with trite Latin and Greek phrases. Fortunately, he responded quickly to medication and was discharged after a brief time.

Many bipolar patients cruise along in a state of controlled excitement or agitation called "hypomania" for extended periods of time. They function at a level of about 6.5 out of a possible 10. It has been said that 50% of the CEOs of large companies are hypomanic. They take risks, they are aggressive, and they work long hours, focusing their excessive mental and emotional energy into feats of productivity that leave regular folks breathless. But without a foundation of psychological strength on which to draw, their frantic efforts can leave them running off the rails in bizarre directions, or crashing helplessly into a black depression.

The following list details the most common symptoms and the frequency of their occurrence in diagnosed manic depression:

Symptoms% of Patients
With Symptoms

Hyperactivity 100
Grandiosity 100
Irritability 100
Mood lability 90
Hyper-sexuality 80 Assaultiveness 75
Distractibility 75
Intrusiveness 60
Somatic complaints 55
Religiosity 50
Regressive behavior (incontinent urinating or defecating) 45
Confusion 35
Ideas of reference 20

(from Kolb, L. C.; Modern Clinical Psychiatry, Philadelphia, W.B. Saunders Co., 1976 p.451)

Patients with bipolar disorder can be some of the most challenging persons to treat. Especially complex are those who cycle between severe mania and then turn around and go into deep depression. Even more complex are the "fast cyclers": those whose highs and lows change by the day or even by the hour!

Alzheimer's Dementia

Our group of students shuffled into the big room joking and pushing, our usual demeanor of cocky sophomores. A hushed queasiness fell over the room as we took in our surroundings. Circling the room above our heads was a sort of broad shelf supporting hundreds of large jars. In each jar was a complete brain.

We were in the Warren State mental hospital and we could hear yelling from some of the patients on the floor above. We became pretty quiet.

"Amyloid"...the tour guide said. "All these brains are from amyloid." In 1972, I had no idea what amyloid was or where it fit in the world of medicine or biochemistry.

It is an amorphous mass of proteins, usually thought to be amassed from immunoglobulins (antibodies and fragments of antibodies) grouped, together. Clumping of amyloid is one of the hallmarks of the brain on autopsy of patients suffering from Alzheimer's dementia.

The clinical features of Alzheimer's dementia features loss of the higher functions of the forebrain -- short-term memory, calculation, judgment and emotions.

The person suffering from Alzheimer's dementia might be able to tell you every person in their third grade class, but not what was said ten minutes ago.

The early features of Alzheimer's dementia often concentrate on anomia: difficulty remembering proper names. An interesting test is to ask the person to name as many items as possible in four categories, each in a one minute time span...vehicles, vegetable, clothing items, and tools. The Alzheimer patient will come up with less than forty every time.

Alzheimer's dementia is very common --3.2% have it in the 70 to 79 age group, and 10.8% in the 80 to 89 group. It definitely increases inexorably with age -- the older one lives, the greater the chance of suffering from this type of dementia.

Recent studies have suggested that the use of aspirin, ibuprofen and other NSAIDS (non-steroidal anti-inflammatory medicines) prevents the development of this disorder. Disease states involving prolonged and chronic inflammation are associated with deposition of amyloid in the tissues. These include tuberculosis, chronic bronchitis, and rheumatoid arthritis. It appears that diseases such as these promote the deposition of amyloid in the tissue when active for many years.

Is it possible that chronic inflammation somewhere in the body can cause Alzheimer's in the brain? This is a tantalizing theory...

Studies indicate that those people that have stimulating hobbies or occupations have a lower risk of Alzheimer's dementia. People with higher education seem to be protected also, although whether there are confounding variables such as poorer health care and increased tobacco use we don't know at this time.

There is a definite genetic disposition of certain forms of Alzheimer's disease, and some very aggressive forms whose gene has been isolated. The genetic transmission of the common variety is not well proven or understood at this time.

Unlike the other mental disorders there is little good treatment for Alzheimer's dementia. The medications available now can slow the progression of the disorder and perhaps delay nursing home admission for a year. But when you think about it, delaying a year is a significant thing for those families dealing with a loved one with Alzheimer's. However, I believe the underlying cause of Alzheimer's dementia will soon be elucidated and those at risk can be identified and the disorder prevented.

Migraine -- Stealer of Days

Thirty-million Americans suffer from migraine headaches and only half seek treatment. That represents a huge number of hours and days wasted, since many people are completely incapacitated during their attacks.

Migraine headaches have a certain pattern. They are throbbing in nature because they arise in the blood vessels surrounding and nourishing the brain. This explains the painful, pulsing nature of the pain that is their trademark. Migraines are usually one-sided, often involving the temple area or eye. They are severe, in that most sufferers describe the pain as "unbearable"- they must isolate themselves, put ice on their heads, and lie down, preferably in a dark, silent room.

Some people experience the well known visual symptoms that precede the migraine. These have been described as sparkles or shimmering lines before the eyes. This represents only 20% of migraine sufferers, and the pattern is called "classic migraines." The rest do not have "flashing lights," and are known as "common migraines."

In 1983, a paper was published in the medical journal *Lancet* by the German researcher Dr. Joseph Egger, exploring the relationship between foods and migraines. In this study, preadolescent boys who were migraine sufferers were placed on a severely restricted diet. The boys were allowed only one kind of meat, vegetable, and fruit for a full week; the purpose being to limit the boys' exposure to stimulating food antigens. The response rate of the boys in eliminating their migraine headaches was...*Ninety three* percent!

Foods were reintroduced to the boys one at a time, to see which foods triggered the migraines. The most common culprits were, in order:

cows' milk 31%
egg 27%
chocolate 25%
orange 24%
wheat 24%
benzoic acid 16%
cheese 16%
tomato 15%
tartrazine 14%

rye 14%
fish 14%
pork 14%
beef 9%
corn 9%

It is important to remember that this list is peculiar to German children in 1983. Children in present day America have a different proportion of allergic foods, with corn and corn products being far higher up the list. This is due to the presence of corn syrup in all infant formulas sold in the United States at this time. These children in Dr. Egger's study also had other symptoms in addition to migraine that resolved during the elimination phase of the study.

These were:
- abdominal pain and gas
- behavior disturbance
- aches in limbs
- fits (seizures)!
- mouth ulcers
- asthma
- eczema

The list above contains some interesting items, but the most fascinating one was seizures ! Who would have thought that eating a food could cause a seizure? Is it possible that Inflammation of the brain can cause most of the severe mental problems of our modern society?[4]

Migraine headache is not a benign process. Studies have shown that migraine sufferers, even in middle age, have twice the rate of stroke as their non migraining counterparts. Since migraine is an inflammatory disease, and chronic inflammation has destructive effects on tissues involved, diet changes and medication to control its effects are essential.

With the exception of seizures, these are symptoms that I see in

---

[4] Is migraine food allergy? A double-blind controlled trial of oligoantigenic diet treatment. Egger J, Carter CM, Wilson J, Turner MW, Soothill JF.
Lancet. 1983 Oct 15;2(8355):865-9.

allergic children every day. There are many papers published in the old days of the 1920s and 1930s referring to epileptic seizures associated with food allergy. This list would suggest that the foods to which the boys were reacting, day in and day out, were affecting other organ systems of the body, not just the blood vessels surrounding the brain.

THE INFLAMED BRAIN

B.R. was a 23–year-old female. She had been institutionalized from the age of 17 to 20 for Schizophrenia. She was on large doses of anti-psychotic medications.. She asked

"I have been reading about gluten sensitivity, and I wonder if it has anything to do with my disorder?"

"There could be, " I answered. " Years ago Dr. Theron Randolph showed a link between food reactions and psychosis. This could be an issue in your case as well."

I instructed her to totally get wheat out of her diet.

She returned a month later, with a vivacity she had not previously exhibited. I said, " Go ahead and reduce your anti-psychotic meds by half.... go slow and let's see how you do."

In two months she was completely off all medications. In a short time she was working full time. She had lost twenty lbs. and was feeling great. She was as strict as strict could be with her diet. Her schizophrenia was being caused by reactions in her intestines.[5]

L. G. was a forty-five-year-old female who'd suffered from migraines and constipation for twenty years. She had at least two debilitating migraines every week. Her life was very difficult.

She came to me one day and asked, "Can I be tested for Celiac disease? My brother was found to have it and maybe this will help my bowel problem!?" We drew some blood and she was positive for all the antibody fragments associated with celiac disease.

Go off all wheat and gluten containing products," I said, "I'm sure you will feel better." She returned two weeks later.

---

[5] Okusaga O, et al, Elevated gliadin antibody levels in individuals with schizophrenia., World J Biol Psychiatry. 2013 Sep;14(7):509-15. doi: 10.3109/15622975.2012.747699. Epub 2013 Jan 3.

She was so excited! Her bowels had become normal with daily bms. Her migraines had decreased by 70% and the remaining ones were not very bad or long-lasting. Researchers in Sheffield, England found lesions in the brains of celiac patients who had suffered for some years, similar to the lesions of multiple sclerosis.[6]

What about Autism.?

We are in an epidemic of this terrible disease. The rate has doubled in the last ten years. This is not due to better diagnosis or changing of definitions.... this is real.

Retrospective studies of children with schizophrenia reveal delays in language acquisition and visual-motor coordination during early childhood before the onset of psychotic symptoms. Alaghband-Rad and colleagues, reviewed the pre-morbid histories of children with COS (childhood onset schizophrenia) and noted language delays and transient motor stereotypies (patterned repetitive movements, postures, and utterances). Their findings suggest early developmental abnormalities of the temporal and frontal lobes as evidenced by pre-psychotic language difficulties; the early transient motor stereotypies indicate developmental abnormalities of the basal ganglia. The similarity of both disorders is striking.

Autism may also be an inflammatory disorder of the brain. Almost all autistic children exhibit signs of immune dysfunction in infancy.... eczema, bowel disturbances, wheezing and chronic ear infections.

A few years ago, Mary Callahan, R.N. wrote a book titled <u>Fighting for Tony.</u> The story of her autistic son and his recovery. In this case, the child was having allergic reactions to cow's milk. His brain was spinning with all the stereotypical behaviors associated with autism.

I have seen this very type of case myself in my own practice. The toddler usually suffers from eczema, chronic ear infections and bowel

---

6   <u>AJNR Am J Neuroradiol.</u> 2010 May;31(5):880-1. doi: 10.3174/ajnr.A1826. Epub 2009 Nov 12.
White matter lesions suggestive of amyotrophic lateral sclerosis attributed to celiac disease.
<u>Brown KJ</u>, <u>Jewells V</u>, <u>Herfarth H</u>, <u>Castillo M</u>.

disturbances in addition to the autistic behaviors.

The offending foods are frequently cow's milk, soy or corn syrup from artificial formulas.

A normal one-year-old will laugh and play peek-a boo, and patty cake, and horsey on the knee till you could drop. The autistic one-year-old will stare at his hand or running water and not interact. It is crucial to identify the autistic child before the age of three, to stop the inflammatory reactions in the brain…. before permanent brain damage results!

The Brain is definitely attached to the rest of the body. The blood brain barrier is really not much of a barrier at all. Reactions, deficiencies and imbalances in the body can cause psychosis, neurosis, depression and autism.

Emotional and psychiatric disorders are common, and that most people suffer from one thing or another at one time or another. There are great new treatments for most. Advances in treatment of mental illness have advanced more in the last twenty years than in all previous recorded history.

The brain is infinitely more complex than any other organ. What combination of chemical or electrical impulses allows you to remember the smell of a rose or picture a fond scene from the past? Neither science nor medicine has an answer. With fantastic complexity comes a wide array of possible derangements, as we have seen. This is okay! What is not okay is to ignore the presence of a problem, deny yourself beneficial treatment, and throw away the opportunity to enjoy the lifestyle and relationships that make us complete and happy.

Last things

The end of a thing is better than the beginning
Ecclesiastes 7:8

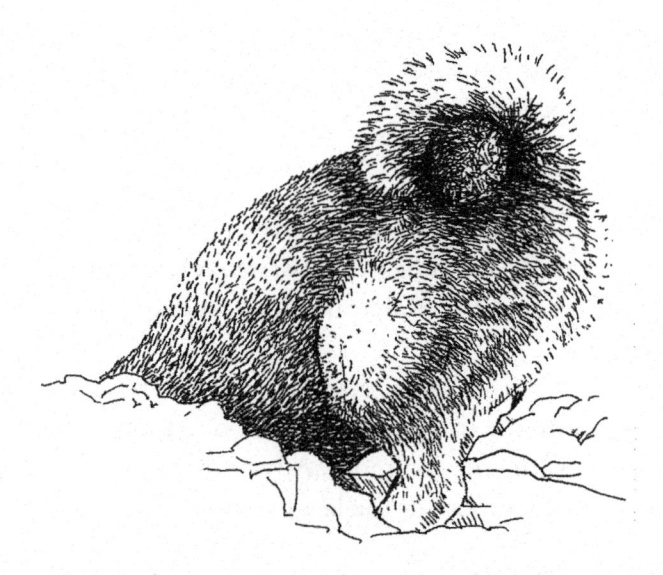

The purpose of this little book is that, perhaps individuals will see themselves and get help and consequently feel better. There is a great deal of untreated disease in this country and unnecessary suffering. Listing the diseases most undiagnosed in the country might look like this:

Sleep apnea - hugely under-recognized and a source of fatigue, high blood pressure, and accidents.

Spastic colon/irritable bowel syndrome- a large pool of patients waiting to be diagnosed.

Bad diets- This might be number one actually. 9 out of 10 Americans could improve their eating habits. Remember , two fruits and two vegetables every day.

High cholesterol- There are millions of people in their 20s, 30s, 40s and 50s who have never had a cholesterol level checked. Those living with high cholesterol are slowly plugging up their arteries year by year. It's really important to know where you fall in this important scheme and to find out what is driving these abnormalities that may lead to an early demise.

Mental illness- So many people are trudging on with depression, anxiety disorders, obsessive compulsive disorder, and others. It would appear that some of most severe illnesses are inflammatory in nature and treatable. *The inflamed brain* is the newest and most important frontier we have Treatment and hope is just waiting for those who care to grab it.

Diabetes mellitus- The ugly step child of our obesity epidemic. There are up to five million undiagnosed diabetics in the United States right now! Many people smolder in a pre-diabetic state for up to ten years before they develop frank diabetes. This can easily be detected by a finger stick glucose check one hour after a meal. If it's over 200 you are diabetic! If it's 160 to 190 you are headed there. Go see your family doctor!

Dementia- Alzheimer's dementia and other dementias are creeping killers not yet fully understood. Some forms are treatable if caught early enough.

Hypothyroidism- One out of ten persons over the age of sixty-five suffers from hidden disease of the thyroid. A common cause of fatigue, it is important to find and to treat.

The annual checkup-
Several articles have appeared in the popular press recently saying things like, "The old annual check-up is over-rated - you won't find

much there and it's not worth the time and money." I disagree- there are several things that should be checked at least annually if you are over forty.

You need to ask your doctor about diet and exercise- how much and what kind is safe and right for you. This is the most important thing possible. Find out what you should weigh and why you don't. This is what is going to keep you going into your old age. It can rescue a sinking unwell older person as well.

Every man and woman over forty should have a yearly rectal exam and test for occult (hidden blood).

A glucose test to check for diabetes or hidden glucose intolerance. Get one no matter when the last meal was...your doctor can work backwards and calculate if you are OK.

A cholesterol test- including subclasses of lipoproteins: HDL, LDL, and triglycerides and the dietary advice to improve them.

You need to have your skin surveyed for skin cancer - to find the ordinary basal cell and squamous cell cancers and to detect the dreaded melanoma.

There is new medical information coming out all the time- you need to ask your doctor about it. Just recently, new data on the slowing of macular degeneration has been released...dietary supplements such as lutein and zinc can help retard that disease. New information regarding hormone replacement in menopausal women and middle aged men is now very big in the news. Each woman must be treated individually, weighing the risks for each possible therapy. How will you ever know unless you ask?

In many ways, I feel that American medicine has lost its way. Concentrating on exotica and expensive and gimmicky tests, while ignoring basic principles- the art of interviewing and preventative medicine and nutrition. Up until recently one half of all medical schools in this country had no formal curriculum for nutrition at all! If you have made it this far in this book you can surmise I firmly believe that all of health depends on diet and exercise. Optimizing yours will determine whether you are vigorous and productive into extreme old age or slip into infirmity prematurely.

Most people go to a doctor only when they are sick. The most foolish words I hear (and I hear them over and over again) is "I wouldn't be here if I wasn't sick." This is usually uttered by people who are obese, diabetic, and quietly growing cancers here and there. That is a shame because your family doctor can be an excellent resource in keeping you healthy, and teaching you to take care of yourself. If your doctor can't picture who you are immediately if you called him at home, you are not seeing him (or her) often enough. *Be somebody!* You'll get much better service for yourself and family members as well.

The quality of your medical services depends on the quality of your relationship with your family doctor. You need to feel comfortable discussing medical, social and mental topics of all kinds with them. That street goes both ways, of course. If your relationship is very superficial, your doctor might not feel comfortable or feel that you are really interested in going deeper into your health, to try to truly optimize your well being. He might not ask you *five questions...*

About The Dogs....

Who can compare in loyalty, intelligence, intuition and unconditional love?